Secrets of the
Infection Control Exam

SECRETS

Study Guide
Your Key to Exam Success

DANB Test Review for the
Infection Control Exam

FREE Study Skills DVD Offer

Dear Customer,

Thank you for your purchase from Mometrix! We consider it an honor and privilege that you have purchased our product and want to ensure your satisfaction.

As a way of showing our appreciation and to help us better serve you, we have developed a Study Skills DVD that we would like to give you for FREE. **This DVD covers our "best practices" for studying for your exam, from using our study materials to preparing for the day of the test.**

All that we ask is that you email us your feedback that would describe your experience so far with our product. Good, bad or indifferent, we want to know what you think!

To get your **FREE Study Skills DVD**, email freedvd@mometrix.com with "FREE STUDY SKILLS DVD" in the subject line and the following information in the body of the email:

   a. The name of the product you purchased.

   b. Your product rating on a scale of 1-5, with 5 being the highest rating.

   c. Your feedback. It can be long, short, or anything in-between, just your impressions and experience so far with our product. Good feedback might include how our study material met your needs and will highlight features of the product that you found helpful.

   d. Your full name and shipping address where you would like us to send your free DVD.

If you have any questions or concerns, please don't hesitate to contact me directly.

Thanks again!

Sincerely,

Jay Willis
Vice President
jay.willis@mometrix.com
1-800-673-8175

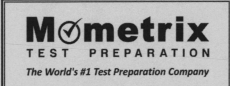

Dear Future Exam Success Story:

First of all, **THANK YOU** for purchasing Mometrix study materials!

Second, congratulations! You are one of the few determined test-takers who are committed to doing whatever it takes to excel on your exam. **You have come to the right place.** We developed these study materials with one goal in mind: to deliver you the information you need in a format that's concise and easy to use.

In addition to optimizing your guide for the content of the test, we've outlined our recommended steps for breaking down the preparation process into small, attainable goals so you can make sure you stay on track.

We've also analyzed the entire test-taking process, identifying the most common pitfalls and showing how you can overcome them and be ready for any curveball the test throws you.

Standardized testing is one of the biggest obstacles on your road to success, which only increases the importance of doing well in the high-pressure, high-stakes environment of test day. Your results on this test could have a significant impact on your future, and this guide provides the information and practical advice to help you achieve your full potential on test day.

Your success is our success

We would love to hear from you! If you would like to share the story of your exam success or if you have any questions or comments in regard to our products, please contact us at **800-673-8175** or **support@mometrix.com**.

Thanks again for your business and we wish you continued success!

Sincerely,
The Mometrix Test Preparation Team

Need more help? Check out our flashcards at: http://MometrixFlashcards.com/DANB

Copyright © 2019 by Mometrix Media LLC. All rights reserved.
Written and edited by the Mometrix Exam Secrets Test Prep Team
Printed in the United States of America

TABLE OF CONTENTS

INTRODUCTION 1

SECRET KEY #1 – PLAN BIG, STUDY SMALL 2
- INFORMATION ORGANIZATION 2
- TIME MANAGEMENT 2
- STUDY ENVIRONMENT 2

SECRET KEY #2 – MAKE YOUR STUDYING COUNT 3
- RETENTION 3
- MODALITY 3

SECRET KEY #3 – PRACTICE THE RIGHT WAY 4
- PRACTICE TEST STRATEGY 5

SECRET KEY #4 – PACE YOURSELF 6

SECRET KEY #5 – HAVE A PLAN FOR GUESSING 7
- WHEN TO START THE GUESSING PROCESS 7
- HOW TO NARROW DOWN THE CHOICES 8
- WHICH ANSWER TO CHOOSE 9

TEST-TAKING STRATEGIES 10
- QUESTION STRATEGIES 10
- ANSWER CHOICE STRATEGIES 11
- GENERAL STRATEGIES 12
- FINAL NOTES 13

STANDARD PRECAUTIONS AND PREVENTION OF DISEASE TRANSMISSION 15
- PATIENT AND DENTAL HEALTHCARE WORKER EDUCATION 15
- DENTAL WATER 29
- THE BODY'S DEFENSE SYSTEM 32
- IMMUNIZATIONS 34
- PREVENTING ADVERSE REACTIONS 37
- STANDARD/UNIVERSAL PRECAUTIONS AND THE PREVENTION OF DISEASE TRANSMISSION ... 38
- PERSONAL PROTECTIVE EQUIPMENT (PPE) 40
- PROTECTING THE PATIENT AND THE OPERATOR 43

PREVENT CROSS-CONTAMINATION DURING PROCEDURES 45

INSTRUMENT/DEVICE PROCESSING 53
- PROCESSING OF REUSABLE DENTAL INSTRUMENTS 53
- MONITORING EQUIPMENT AND STERILIZERS 60

OCCUPATIONAL SAFETY/ADMINISTRATIVE PROCEDURES 62
- OCCUPATIONAL SAFETY 62
- STANDARDS AND PROTOCOLS 64

DANB PRACTICE TEST 76

ANSWER KEY AND EXPLANATIONS 84

HOW TO OVERCOME TEST ANXIETY 94
- CAUSES OF TEST ANXIETY 94
- ELEMENTS OF TEST ANXIETY 95
- EFFECTS OF TEST ANXIETY 95

    Physical Steps for Beating Test Anxiety 96
    Mental Steps for Beating Test Anxiety 97
    Study Strategy 98
    Test Tips 100
    Important Qualification 101

THANK YOU 102

ADDITIONAL BONUS MATERIAL 103

Introduction

Thank you for purchasing this resource! You have made the choice to prepare yourself for a test that could have a huge impact on your future, and this guide is designed to help you be fully ready for test day. Obviously, it's important to have a solid understanding of the test material, but you also need to be prepared for the unique environment and stressors of the test, so that you can perform to the best of your abilities.

For this purpose, the first section that appears in this guide is the **Secret Keys**. We've devoted countless hours to meticulously researching what works and what doesn't, and we've boiled down our findings to the five most impactful steps you can take to improve your performance on the test. We start at the beginning with study planning and move through the preparation process, all the way to the testing strategies that will help you get the most out of what you know when you're finally sitting in front of the test.

We recommend that you start preparing for your test as far in advance as possible. However, if you've bought this guide as a last-minute study resource and only have a few days before your test, we recommend that you skip over the first two Secret Keys since they address a long-term study plan.

If you struggle with **test anxiety**, we strongly encourage you to check out our recommendations for how you can overcome it. Test anxiety is a formidable foe, but it can be beaten, and we want to make sure you have the tools you need to defeat it.

Secret Key #1 – Plan Big, Study Small

There's a lot riding on your performance. If you want to ace this test, you're going to need to keep your skills sharp and the material fresh in your mind. You need a plan that lets you review everything you need to know while still fitting in your schedule. We'll break this strategy down into three categories.

Information Organization

Start with the information you already have: the official test outline. From this, you can make a complete list of all the concepts you need to cover before the test. Organize these concepts into groups that can be studied together, and create a list of any related vocabulary you need to learn so you can brush up on any difficult terms. You'll want to keep this vocabulary list handy once you actually start studying since you may need to add to it along the way.

Time Management

Once you have your set of study concepts, decide how to spread them out over the time you have left before the test. Break your study plan into small, clear goals so you have a manageable task for each day and know exactly what you're doing. Then just focus on one small step at a time. When you manage your time this way, you don't need to spend hours at a time studying. Studying a small block of content for a short period each day helps you retain information better and avoid stressing over how much you have left to do. You can relax knowing that you have a plan to cover everything in time. In order for this strategy to be effective though, you have to start studying early and stick to your schedule. Avoid the exhaustion and futility that comes from last-minute cramming!

Study Environment

The environment you study in has a big impact on your learning. Studying in a coffee shop, while probably more enjoyable, is not likely to be as fruitful as studying in a quiet room. It's important to keep distractions to a minimum. You're only planning to study for a short block of time, so make the most of it. Don't pause to check your phone or get up to find a snack. It's also important to **avoid multitasking**. Research has consistently shown that multitasking will make your studying dramatically less effective. Your study area should also be comfortable and well-lit so you don't have the distraction of straining your eyes or sitting on an uncomfortable chair.

The time of day you study is also important. You want to be rested and alert. Don't wait until just before bedtime. Study when you'll be most likely to comprehend and remember. Even better, if you know what time of day your test will be, set that time aside for study. That way your brain will be used to working on that subject at that specific time and you'll have a better chance of recalling information.

Finally, it can be helpful to team up with others who are studying for the same test. Your actual studying should be done in as isolated an environment as possible, but the work of organizing the information and setting up the study plan can be divided up. In between study sessions, you can discuss with your teammates the concepts that you're all studying and quiz each other on the details. Just be sure that your teammates are as serious about the test as you are. If you find that your study time is being replaced with social time, you might need to find a new team.

Secret Key #2 – Make Your Studying Count

You're devoting a lot of time and effort to preparing for this test, so you want to be absolutely certain it will pay off. This means doing more than just reading the content and hoping you can remember it on test day. It's important to make every minute of study count. There are two main areas you can focus on to make your studying count:

Retention

It doesn't matter how much time you study if you can't remember the material. You need to make sure you are retaining the concepts. To check your retention of the information you're learning, try recalling it at later times with minimal prompting. Try carrying around flashcards and glance at one or two from time to time or ask a friend who's also studying for the test to quiz you.

To enhance your retention, look for ways to put the information into practice so that you can apply it rather than simply recalling it. If you're using the information in practical ways, it will be much easier to remember. Similarly, it helps to solidify a concept in your mind if you're not only reading it to yourself but also explaining it to someone else. Ask a friend to let you teach them about a concept you're a little shaky on (or speak aloud to an imaginary audience if necessary). As you try to summarize, define, give examples, and answer your friend's questions, you'll understand the concepts better and they will stay with you longer. Finally, step back for a big picture view and ask yourself how each piece of information fits with the whole subject. When you link the different concepts together and see them working together as a whole, it's easier to remember the individual components.

Finally, practice showing your work on any multi-step problems, even if you're just studying. Writing out each step you take to solve a problem will help solidify the process in your mind, and you'll be more likely to remember it during the test.

Modality

Modality simply refers to the means or method by which you study. Choosing a study modality that fits your own individual learning style is crucial. No two people learn best in exactly the same way, so it's important to know your strengths and use them to your advantage.

For example, if you learn best by visualization, focus on visualizing a concept in your mind and draw an image or a diagram. Try color-coding your notes, illustrating them, or creating symbols that will trigger your mind to recall a learned concept. If you learn best by hearing or discussing information, find a study partner who learns the same way or read aloud to yourself. Think about how to put the information in your own words. Imagine that you are giving a lecture on the topic and record yourself so you can listen to it later.

For any learning style, flashcards can be helpful. Organize the information so you can take advantage of spare moments to review. Underline key words or phrases. Use different colors for different categories. Mnemonic devices (such as creating a short list in which every item starts with the same letter) can also help with retention. Find what works best for you and use it to store the information in your mind most effectively and easily.

Secret Key #3 – Practice the Right Way

Your success on test day depends not only on how many hours you put into preparing, but also on whether you prepared the right way. It's good to check along the way to see if your studying is paying off. One of the most effective ways to do this is by taking practice tests to evaluate your progress. Practice tests are useful because they show exactly where you need to improve. Every time you take a practice test, pay special attention to these three groups of questions:

- The questions you got wrong
- The questions you had to guess on, even if you guessed right
- The questions you found difficult or slow to work through

This will show you exactly what your weak areas are, and where you need to devote more study time. Ask yourself why each of these questions gave you trouble. Was it because you didn't understand the material? Was it because you didn't remember the vocabulary? Do you need more repetitions on this type of question to build speed and confidence? Dig into those questions and figure out how you can strengthen your weak areas as you go back to review the material.

Additionally, many practice tests have a section explaining the answer choices. It can be tempting to read the explanation and think that you now have a good understanding of the concept. However, an explanation likely only covers part of the question's broader context. Even if the explanation makes sense, **go back and investigate** every concept related to the question until you're positive you have a thorough understanding.

As you go along, keep in mind that the practice test is just that: practice. Memorizing these questions and answers will not be very helpful on the actual test because it is unlikely to have any of the same exact questions. If you only know the right answers to the sample questions, you won't be prepared for the real thing. **Study the concepts** until you understand them fully, and then you'll be able to answer any question that shows up on the test.

It's important to wait on the practice tests until you're ready. If you take a test on your first day of study, you may be overwhelmed by the amount of material covered and how much you need to learn. Work up to it gradually.

On test day, you'll need to be prepared for answering questions, managing your time, and using the test-taking strategies you've learned. It's a lot to balance, like a mental marathon that will have a big impact on your future. Like training for a marathon, you'll need to start slowly and work your way up. When test day arrives, you'll be ready.

Start with the strategies you've read in the first two Secret Keys—plan your course and study in the way that works best for you. If you have time, consider using multiple study resources to get different approaches to the same concepts. It can be helpful to see difficult concepts from more than one angle. Then find a good source for practice tests. Many times, the test website will suggest potential study resources or provide sample tests.

Practice Test Strategy

When you're ready to start taking practice tests, follow this strategy:

1. Take the first test with no time constraints and with your notes and study guide handy. Take your time and focus on applying the strategies you've learned.
2. Take the second practice test open-book as well, but set a timer and practice pacing yourself to finish in time.
3. Take any other practice tests as if it were test day. Set a timer and put away your study materials. Sit at a table or desk in a quiet room, imagine yourself at the testing center, and answer questions as quickly and accurately as possible.
4. Keep repeating step 3 on a regular basis until you run out of practice tests or it's time for the actual test. Your mind will be ready for the schedule and stress of test day, and you'll be able to focus on recalling the material you've learned.

Secret Key #4 – Pace Yourself

Once you're fully prepared for the material on the test, your biggest challenge on test day will be managing your time. Just knowing that the clock is ticking can make you panic even if you have plenty of time left. Work on pacing yourself so you can build confidence against the time constraints of the exam. Pacing is a difficult skill to master, especially in a high-pressure environment, so **practice is vital**.

Set time expectations for your pace based on how much time is available. For example, if a section has 60 questions and the time limit is 30 minutes, you know you have to average 30 seconds or less per question in order to answer them all. Although 30 seconds is the hard limit, set 25 seconds per question as your goal, so you reserve extra time to spend on harder questions. When you budget extra time for the harder questions, you no longer have any reason to stress when those questions take longer to answer.

Don't let this time expectation distract you from working through the test at a calm, steady pace, but keep it in mind so you don't spend too much time on any one question. Recognize that taking extra time on one question you don't understand may keep you from answering two that you do understand later in the test. If your time limit for a question is up and you're still not sure of the answer, mark it and move on, and come back to it later if the time and the test format allow. If the testing format doesn't allow you to return to earlier questions, just make an educated guess; then put it out of your mind and move on.

On the easier questions, be careful not to rush. It may seem wise to hurry through them so you have more time for the challenging ones, but it's not worth missing one if you know the concept and just didn't take the time to read the question fully. Work efficiently but make sure you understand the question and have looked at all of the answer choices, since more than one may seem right at first.

Even if you're paying attention to the time, you may find yourself a little behind at some point. You should speed up to get back on track, but do so wisely. Don't panic; just take a few seconds less on each question until you're caught up. Don't guess without thinking, but do look through the answer choices and eliminate any you know are wrong. If you can get down to two choices, it is often worthwhile to guess from those. Once you've chosen an answer, move on and don't dwell on any that you skipped or had to hurry through. If a question was taking too long, chances are it was one of the harder ones, so you weren't as likely to get it right anyway.

On the other hand, if you find yourself getting ahead of schedule, it may be beneficial to slow down a little. The more quickly you work, the more likely you are to make a careless mistake that will affect your score. You've budgeted time for each question, so don't be afraid to spend that time. Practice an efficient but careful pace to get the most out of the time you have.

Secret Key #5 – Have a Plan for Guessing

When you're taking the test, you may find yourself stuck on a question. Some of the answer choices seem better than others, but you don't see the one answer choice that is obviously correct. What do you do?

The scenario described above is very common, yet most test takers have not effectively prepared for it. Developing and practicing a plan for guessing may be one of the single most effective uses of your time as you get ready for the exam.

In developing your plan for guessing, there are three questions to address:

- When should you start the guessing process?
- How should you narrow down the choices?
- Which answer should you choose?

When to Start the Guessing Process

Unless your plan for guessing is to select C every time (which, despite its merits, is not what we recommend), you need to leave yourself enough time to apply your answer elimination strategies. Since you have a limited amount of time for each question, that means that if you're going to give yourself the best shot at guessing correctly, you have to decide quickly whether or not you will guess.

Of course, the best-case scenario is that you don't have to guess at all, so first, see if you can answer the question based on your knowledge of the subject and basic reasoning skills. Focus on the key words in the question and try to jog your memory of related topics. Give yourself a chance to bring the knowledge to mind, but once you realize that you don't have (or you can't access) the knowledge you need to answer the question, it's time to start the guessing process.

It's almost always better to start the guessing process too early than too late. It only takes a few seconds to remember something and answer the question from knowledge. Carefully eliminating wrong answer choices takes longer. Plus, going through the process of eliminating answer choices can actually help jog your memory.

Summary: Start the guessing process as soon as you decide that you can't answer the question based on your knowledge.

How to Narrow Down the Choices

The next chapter in this book (**Test-Taking Strategies**) includes a wide range of strategies for how to approach questions and how to look for answer choices to eliminate. You will definitely want to read those carefully, practice them, and figure out which ones work best for you. Here though, we're going to address a mindset rather than a particular strategy.

Your chances of guessing an answer correctly depend on how many options you are choosing from.

How many choices you have	How likely you are to guess correctly
5	20%
4	25%
3	33%
2	50%
1	100%

You can see from this chart just how valuable it is to be able to eliminate incorrect answers and make an educated guess, but there are two things that many test takers do that cause them to miss out on the benefits of guessing:

- Accidentally eliminating the correct answer
- Selecting an answer based on an impression

We'll look at the first one here, and the second one in the next section.

To avoid accidentally eliminating the correct answer, we recommend a thought exercise called **the $5 challenge**. In this challenge, you only eliminate an answer choice from contention if you are willing to bet $5 on it being wrong. Why $5? Five dollars is a small but not insignificant amount of money. It's an amount you could afford to lose but wouldn't want to throw away. And while losing $5 once might not hurt too much, doing it twenty times will set you back $100. In the same way, each small decision you make—eliminating a choice here, guessing on a question there—won't by itself impact your score very much, but when you put them all together, they can make a big difference. By holding each answer choice elimination decision to a higher standard, you can reduce the risk of accidentally eliminating the correct answer.

The $5 challenge can also be applied in a positive sense: If you are willing to bet $5 that an answer choice *is* correct, go ahead and mark it as correct.

Summary: Only eliminate an answer choice if you are willing to bet $5 that it is wrong.

Which Answer to Choose

You're taking the test. You've run into a hard question and decided you'll have to guess. You've eliminated all the answer choices you're willing to bet $5 on. Now you have to pick an answer. Why do we even need to talk about this? Why can't you just pick whichever one you feel like when the time comes?

The answer to these questions is that if you don't come into the test with a plan, you'll rely on your impression to select an answer choice, and if you do that, you risk falling into a trap. The test writers know that everyone who takes their test will be guessing on some of the questions, so they intentionally write wrong answer choices to seem plausible. You still have to pick an answer though, and if the wrong answer choices are designed to look right, how can you ever be sure that you're not falling for their trap? The best solution we've found to this dilemma is to take the decision out of your hands entirely. Here is the process we recommend:

Once you've eliminated any choices that you are confident (willing to bet $5) are wrong, select the first remaining choice as your answer.

Whether you choose to select the first remaining choice, the second, or the last, the important thing is that you use some preselected standard. Using this approach guarantees that you will not be enticed into selecting an answer choice that looks right, because you are not basing your decision on how the answer choices look.

This is not meant to make you question your knowledge. Instead, it is to help you recognize the difference between your knowledge and your impressions. There's a huge difference between thinking an answer is right because of what you know, and thinking an answer is right because it looks or sounds like it should be right.

Summary: To ensure that your selection is appropriately random, make a predetermined selection from among all answer choices you have not eliminated.

Test-Taking Strategies

This section contains a list of test-taking strategies that you may find helpful as you work through the test. By taking what you know and applying logical thought, you can maximize your chances of answering any question correctly!

It is very important to realize that every question is different and every person is different: no single strategy will work on every question, and no single strategy will work for every person. That's why we've included all of them here, so you can try them out and determine which ones work best for different types of questions and which ones work best for you.

Question Strategies

Read Carefully

Read the question and answer choices carefully. Don't miss the question because you misread the terms. You have plenty of time to read each question thoroughly and make sure you understand what is being asked. Yet a happy medium must be attained, so don't waste too much time. You must read carefully, but efficiently.

Contextual Clues

Look for contextual clues. If the question includes a word you are not familiar with, look at the immediate context for some indication of what the word might mean. Contextual clues can often give you all the information you need to decipher the meaning of an unfamiliar word. Even if you can't determine the meaning, you may be able to narrow down the possibilities enough to make a solid guess at the answer to the question.

Prefixes

If you're having trouble with a word in the question or answer choices, try dissecting it. Take advantage of every clue that the word might include. Prefixes and suffixes can be a huge help. Usually they allow you to determine a basic meaning. Pre- means before, post- means after, pro - is positive, de- is negative. From prefixes and suffixes, you can get an idea of the general meaning of the word and try to put it into context.

Hedge Words

Watch out for critical hedge words, such as *likely, may, can, sometimes, often, almost, mostly, usually, generally, rarely,* and *sometimes*. Question writers insert these hedge phrases to cover every possibility. Often an answer choice will be wrong simply because it leaves no room for exception. Be on guard for answer choices that have definitive words such as *exactly* and *always*.

Switchback Words

Stay alert for *switchbacks*. These are the words and phrases frequently used to alert you to shifts in thought. The most common switchback words are *but, although,* and *however*. Others include *nevertheless, on the other hand, even though, while, in spite of, despite, regardless of*. Switchback words are important to catch because they can change the direction of the question or an answer choice.

Face Value

When in doubt, use common sense. Accept the situation in the problem at face value. Don't read too much into it. These problems will not require you to make wild assumptions. If you have to go beyond creativity and warp time or space in order to have an answer choice fit the question, then you should move on and consider the other answer choices. These are normal problems rooted in reality. The applicable relationship or explanation may not be readily apparent, but it is there for you to figure out. Use your common sense to interpret anything that isn't clear.

Answer Choice Strategies

Answer Selection

The most thorough way to pick an answer choice is to identify and eliminate wrong answers until only one is left, then confirm it is the correct answer. Sometimes an answer choice may immediately seem right, but be careful. The test writers will usually put more than one reasonable answer choice on each question, so take a second to read all of them and make sure that the other choices are not equally obvious. As long as you have time left, it is better to read every answer choice than to pick the first one that looks right without checking the others.

Answer Choice Families

An answer choice family consists of two (in rare cases, three) answer choices that are very similar in construction and cannot all be true at the same time. If you see two answer choices that are direct opposites or parallels, one of them is usually the correct answer. For instance, if one answer choice says that quantity x increases and another either says that quantity x decreases (opposite) or says that quantity y increases (parallel), then those answer choices would fall into the same family. An answer choice that doesn't match the construction of the answer choice family is more likely to be incorrect. Most questions will not have answer choice families, but when they do appear, you should be prepared to recognize them.

Eliminate Answers

Eliminate answer choices as soon as you realize they are wrong, but make sure you consider all possibilities. If you are eliminating answer choices and realize that the last one you are left with is also wrong, don't panic. Start over and consider each choice again. There may be something you missed the first time that you will realize on the second pass.

Avoid Fact Traps

Don't be distracted by an answer choice that is factually true but doesn't answer the question. You are looking for the choice that answers the question. Stay focused on what the question is asking for so you don't accidentally pick an answer that is true but incorrect. Always go back to the question and make sure the answer choice you've selected actually answers the question and is not merely a true statement.

Extreme Statements

In general, you should avoid answers that put forth extreme actions as standard practice or proclaim controversial ideas as established fact. An answer choice that states the "process should be used in certain situations, if..." is much more likely to be correct than one that states the "process should be discontinued completely." The first is a calm rational statement and doesn't even make a definitive, uncompromising stance, using a hedge word *if* to provide wiggle room, whereas the second choice is a radical idea and far more extreme.

Benchmark

As you read through the answer choices and you come across one that seems to answer the question well, mentally select that answer choice. This is not your final answer, but it's the one that will help you evaluate the other answer choices. The one that you selected is your benchmark or standard for judging each of the other answer choices. Every other answer choice must be compared to your benchmark. That choice is correct until proven otherwise by another answer choice beating it. If you find a better answer, then that one becomes your new benchmark. Once you've decided that no other choice answers the question as well as your benchmark, you have your final answer.

Predict the Answer

Before you even start looking at the answer choices, it is often best to try to predict the answer. When you come up with the answer on your own, it is easier to avoid distractions and traps because you will know exactly what to look for. The right answer choice is unlikely to be word-for-word what you came up with, but it should be a close match. Even if you are confident that you have the right answer, you should still take the time to read each option before moving on.

General Strategies

Tough Questions

If you are stumped on a problem or it appears too hard or too difficult, don't waste time. Move on! Remember though, if you can quickly check for obviously incorrect answer choices, your chances of guessing correctly are greatly improved. Before you completely give up, at least try to knock out a couple of possible answers. Eliminate what you can and then guess at the remaining answer choices before moving on.

Check Your Work

Since you will probably not know every term listed and the answer to every question, it is important that you get credit for the ones that you do know. Don't miss any questions through careless mistakes. If at all possible, try to take a second to look back over your answer selection and make sure you've selected the correct answer choice and haven't made a costly careless mistake (such as marking an answer choice that you didn't mean to mark). This quick double check should more than pay for itself in caught mistakes for the time it costs.

Pace Yourself

It's easy to be overwhelmed when you're looking at a page full of questions; your mind is confused and full of random thoughts, and the clock is ticking down faster than you would like. Calm down and maintain the pace that you have set for yourself. Especially as you get down to the last few minutes of the test, don't let the small numbers on the clock make you panic. As long as you are on track by monitoring your pace, you are guaranteed to have time for each question.

Don't Rush

It is very easy to make errors when you are in a hurry. Maintaining a fast pace in answering questions is pointless if it makes you miss questions that you would have gotten right otherwise. Test writers like to include distracting information and wrong answers that seem right. Taking a little extra time to avoid careless mistakes can make all the difference in your test score. Find a pace that allows you to be confident in the answers that you select.

Keep Moving

Panicking will not help you pass the test, so do your best to stay calm and keep moving. Taking deep breaths and going through the answer elimination steps you practiced can help to break through a stress barrier and keep your pace.

Final Notes

The combination of a solid foundation of content knowledge and the confidence that comes from practicing your plan for applying that knowledge is the key to maximizing your performance on test day. As your foundation of content knowledge is built up and strengthened, you'll find that the strategies included in this chapter become more and more effective in helping you quickly sift through the distractions and traps of the test to isolate the correct answer.

Now it's time to move on to the test content chapters of this book, but be sure to keep your goal in mind. As you read, think about how you will be able to apply this information on the test. If you've already seen sample questions for the test and you have an idea of the question format and style, try to come up with questions of your own that you can answer based on what you're reading. This will give you valuable practice applying your knowledge in the same ways you can expect to on test day.

Good luck and good studying!

Standard Precautions and Prevention of Disease Transmission

Patient and Dental Healthcare Worker Education

Infection control

Reasoning behind practicing infection control in dental setting

Infection control should be practiced in the dental setting to deter transmission and disease development at any point and in any direction. Infectious agents can be spread from the patient to members of the dental team and vice versa, between patients, from the dental office into the community, and from the outside community to the patients. The main pathway of cross-contamination from patient to members of the dental team is from the patient's mouth, either through direct contact via skin breaks, droplet infection (through inhalation, skin breaks, or mucosal contact), or indirect contact via cuts or punctures. Similarly, the main patient-to-patient or office-to-community means of transmission are via the mouth through indirect contact. The dental team can transmit infections to the patient's mouth directly through hand lesions or bleeding or indirectly on instruments. They can also contaminate the patient by droplet infection through inhalation or contact with oral mucosa. The main way dental workers transmit infections to their family is through intimate contact with bodily fluids, and the primary community to patient mode is direct contact with contaminated municipal water.

Main goal

The main goal of infection control measures is to decrease the dose of microorganisms that may be transmitted between people or between individuals and surfaces. There are a variety of measures that serve this goal, discussed further elsewhere. The end result of exposure to an infectious agent is dependent on three interrelated factors defined as follows:

Presence of health or disease = (virulence of the infectious agent x its dose)/resistance of the host

If the infectious agent is of low virulence and low exposure dose and the individual has good defense mechanisms and high resistance, health is favored over disease. Conversely, a highly virulent microorganism administered at high dose to a person with low resistance will most likely result in disease. Virulence is an inherent property of each species of microorganism and host resistance is hard to control, so the factor that can be regulated is exposure dose.

Special considerations during office remodeling or construction

One of the biggest concerns during office remodeling or construction is the potential environmental dissemination of microorganisms resulting in nosocomial infections. Nosocomial infections are those acquired while in a hospital or other medical facility such as a dental office. Construction activity creates additional moisture and water in the area, which creates a favorable environment for certain microorganisms. Some of the most common construction-related infectious outbreaks involve fungi like *Aspergillus* or bacteria such as Group A *Streptococcus* or *Pseudomonas*. It is crucial to keep construction activity as isolated from patient care areas as possible, and provisional barriers may need to be constructed between the two. Contractors are responsible for cleaning their working zones, but non-construction areas will need to be cleaned more often and more comprehensively. Extra precautions for both employees and patients are generally needed, and certain types of patients may need to rescheduled until after completion of the construction work (for example those with respiratory problems).

Infectious disease

Steps in development

There are basically 6 steps in the development of an infectious disease. The first two are some source of the microorganism and the subsequent escape of it from the source. Escape routes include coughing, talking, and removal of anything that has been in the mouth (instruments, x-ray film, etc.). An infectious disease can also escape in droplets or aerosols generated through equipment use. The next step is the transmission of the agent to a new individual through direct contact such as at the mouth, indirect contact with anything that has been contaminated (for example surfaces, hands or sharps), contact with large droplets that are sprayed or splattered, or inhalation of smaller airborne droplets or aerosol particles. Further development of the infectious disease includes entry of the agent into the new person (through inhalation, ingestion, contact with mucous membranes, or through breaks in the skin), the infection phase in which the microorganism endures and multiplies in or on the body, and lastly, causation of some type of harmful bodily damage.

Stages

Infectious diseases have 4 stages. The first is the incubation stage, which is the time from when the infectious agent entered the body until symptoms of disease are evident. The length of this stage is extremely variable depending on the disease, ranging, for example, from several days for influenza to a decade or more for HIV. After the incubation period is a prodromal stage, which is when initial symptoms such as malaise or headache come into view. As symptoms progress and the person becomes visibly sick, he or she enters the acute stage. This is the period with the most potential for transmission of the agent when dental visits should be avoided if possible. The last stage is generally the convalescent or recovery stage in which the microbe levels are decreases and detrimental microbial products are being deactivated by the body. Transmission is still possible, however, as the infectious agent has not been entirely eradicated. Again the length of convalescence is quite variable depending on the agent and some diseases are chronic. During any stage, some people appear asymptomatic but are still carriers.

Bloodborne diseases

Bloodborne diseases are any diseases that can be transmitted via the blood or other bodily fluids, such as semen, mother's milk, or saliva. Saliva is deemed potentially infectious because bleeding can release bloodborne pathogens into the fluid. The bloodborne diseases of particular interest to the dental worker are viral hepatitis (particularly the form transmitted by hepatitis B virus (HBV), which is extremely virulent) and human immunodeficiency virus (HIV), which can develop into acquired immunodeficiency syndrome (AIDS). AIDS is currently manageable but not eradicable. Other bacterial and viral diseases can also be spread via the blood or bodily fluids.

Hepatitis viruses spread via fecal-oral routes

The two main hepatitis viruses spread via fecal or oral routes are hepatitis A virus and hepatitis E virus. Since neither has been demonstrated to be transmitted via blood or bodily fluids, they do not present particular risks for dental workers. Neither exists chronically in carrier states or has any possible sequelae. Both have acute onsets starting about 15 days to several months after exposure. Hepatitis A virus (HAV) is a non-enveloped single-stranded RNA picornavirus. Acute infections almost never result in death. There is an available vaccine for HAV (usually suggested for those traveling to countries with inadequate sanitation) as well as antibody screening tests. The latter include anti-HAV, antibody to HAV, which can be found at onset of symptoms and endures throughout life, and IgM anti-HAV, which detects the IgM class of antibodies only present after recent infection.

Hepatitis E virus (HEV) is a non-enveloped, single-stranded RNA calicivirus. There are no vaccines for protection against HEV and no available tests to detect anti-HEV, antibody to HEV, which theoretically would indicate exposure. Contraction of HEV during pregnancy can prove fatal.

Transmission of HIV

Human immunodeficiency virus, HIV, is a bloodborne disease. It is transmitted through exposure to HIV-positive blood, through sexual contact, or perinatally from mother to child. Excellent screening tests for anti-HIV and other characteristic proteins such as p24 now make the likelihood of exposure through blood transfusions practically nonexistent. However, other high-risk practices, such as sharing of injection needles by intravenous drug users, account for about a quarter of cases. HIV has been identified in other bodily fluids, including saliva. The largest source of HIV infection is transmission through unprotected sexual practices with an HIV-positive individual. HIV can also be passed across the placenta perinatally from mother to child or occasionally via breast milk. This transmission can be dramatically diminished through drug therapy during pregnancy.

Systemic diseases that have oral lesions

Syphilis, caused by the spirochete *Treponema pallidum,* can initially show up as an open ulcer on the tongue or lip. However, it is a systemic disease, and if left untreated, can result in secondary patches on the mucous membranes of the oral cavity about 2-10 weeks after the initial lesion. The two main systemic viral diseases that can result in oral lesions are chickenpox and infectious mononucleosis. The causative agent of chicken pox (as well as shingles in older individuals) is human herpesvirus type 3, also known as vermicelli zoster virus. It is transmitted by droplet infection to the respiratory tract, the bloodstream, and eventually to the skin and other organs, possibly manifesting orally as vesicles. Another herpes virus, HHV-4 or Epstein-Barr virus, is the causative agent of infectious mononucleosis, which is transmitted by contact with saliva or sometimes through blood transfusions. The infected individual generally has a fever and fatigue and may have a number of oral manifestations, such as sore throat, oral ulcers, red areas in the palate called petechiae, whitish tongue lesions called hairy leukoplakia, and a number of cancers.

Bacterial diseases transmitted by respiratory and oral fluids

Various species of streptococcus cause respiratory diseases. Pharyngitis and scarlet fever are spread via droplets containing *Streptococcus pyogenes* (discussed further on another card). Pneumonia, inflammation of the lung, can be caused by a number of bacteria or viruses, including *Streptococcus pneumoniae*. *S. pneumoniae* is transmitted via respiratory/oral droplets, is prevalent asymptomatically in a large number of children and adults. The bacterium can also cause middle ear infections, meningitis, and sinusitis. Pneumonia can also be caused by other agents, such as *Staphylococcus aureus* and *Haemophilus influenzae*. The latter can produce meningitis, sinusitis, conjunctivitis, and bronchitis. Other bacterial respiratory diseases of interest are diphtheria with *Corynebacterium diphtheriae* as the causative agent and meningitis caused by *Neisseria meningitides*. *C. diphtheriae* is generally not a problem as it, along with agents for pertusis (whopping cough) and tetanus (lockjaw, causative agent *Clostridium tetani*), is included in the DPT vaccine given to children.

Viral diseases transmitted via respiratory/oral fluids

Some forms of pneumonia are viral in origin, including influenza virus, adenovirus, and respiratory syncytial virus. The common cold is caused by any number of possible rhinoviruses plus other viral agents. There are a number of influenza viruses that can bring about influenza (fever, sore throat, headache, dry cough, muscle pain, etc.), bronchitis, and pneumonia. Several human herpesviruses can have respiratory manifestations. Chickenpox (HHV-3) can be spread by airborne droplets, and herpesviruses types 5, 6, and 7 have all been demonstrated in saliva, possibly causing CMV, cytomegalovirus disease, and roseola respectively. The herpesviruses may also have unknown consequences. HHV-4 or Epstein Barr virus is the causative agent of infectious mononucleosis as well. Measles (rubeola), rubella, and mumps can all be transmitted by inhaled respiratory/oral droplets; the MMR vaccine given to children provides protection against all three. Measles is characterized by rash and fever, rubella by rash on the face and often elsewhere, and mumps by swelling of the salivary glands.

Infection control procedures for each mode of transmission

Briefly, the means of controlling the possibility of disease transmission are as follows:

1. Patient to dental team - Overall measures used by the dental team consist of hand washing, gloves, other personal protective equipment, rubber dams (for droplet infection protection), and immunization. In addition, indirect contact can be prevented with recommended needle safety and cleanup procedures.
2. Dental team to patient - Transmission can be avoided by the use of hand washing, gloves, immunization, instrument sterilization, surface disinfection, and masks and face shields (for droplet infection protection) by the dental team.
3. Patient to patient - As this type of transmission is mainly through indirect contact, infection control procedures include things like sterilization of instruments, disinfection of surfaces, flushing of dental unit water lines, changing of personal protective equipment when needed, and use of disposables.
4. Office to community - Preventing spread of disease from the office to the community requires measures such as proper handling of waste and contaminated laundry.
5. Dental team to family - The dental team can protect family members by immunization.
6. Community to patient - Preventing the spread of disease from community to patient requires good water control procedures.

Biochemical components of microbes

Categories of microbes include bacteria, viruses, fungi and protozoa. Each has a different structure, but these microbes share many of the same biochemical macromolecules. All microorganisms carry their genetic information through their DNA (deoxyribonucleic acid) and/or RNA (ribonucleic acid) as do humans and other organisms. They contain protein composed of amino acids utilized as structural components (cell walls, cytoplasm membranes, flagella in bacteria; capsids and envelope proteins in viruses) or enzymes acting as biochemical catalysts. Microorganisms also contain polysaccharides and lipids. Polysaccharides are made up of monosaccharides or sugars such as glucose and fructose and are found in structures such as capsules or storage granules. They can be complexed to proteins as glycoproteins, which are found in things such as surface projections on bacteria called fimbriae or as components of viral envelopes. Lipids are made up of fatty acids and glycerol and are found in structures like bacterial cytoplasm membranes and viral envelopes. They are associated with proteins as lipoproteins in cell walls and with polysaccharides as lipopolysaccharides such as endotoxins in some bacteria.

Bacteria

Determining types

Bacteria are designated by their genus and species within that genus. They are tiny (micrometer range), single cell organisms. Each type of bacterium has a characteristic size and shape visible microscopically (known as cell morphology), a typical staining pattern, distinctive colony growth on agar media, certain metabolic properties, distinguishing antibodies on their surface that elicit immunological responses, and species-specific genetic potential expressed on their DNA and RNA. All bacteria are either spherical, rod-shaped, or spiral, termed cocci, bacilli, or spirilla respectively; cocci and bacilli may exist in clusters or chains. The most common staining method used is called a gram stain, which differentiates all bacteria as either gram-positive (blue or purple) or gram-negative (red).

Unique structures

In gram-negative bacteria, there is an outer membrane containing endotoxin surrounding the cell wall. Endotoxin, which is a lip polysaccharide-protein complex, can be discharged after cell death and cause various untoward reactions in the host. Some bacteria have capsules outside the cell wall (gram-positive) or outer membrane (gram-negative). Capsules, which contain polysaccharides (possibly in conjunction with proteins) and water, are generated by the cytoplasmic membrane and aid in functions such as surface attachment, defense against phagocytosis by the host, and protection against drying. Certain bacteria have proteinaceous threads projecting outward called flagella, which aid in locomotion. Many bacteria have fimbriae (also known as pili), which are short projections that make it easier for the bacterium to attach to surfaces and transport DNA between cells. Bacteria with pili tend to be more virulent because they can attach more easily to their host. Another means of increased virulence found in some bacteria is endospore or spore production. Spores are found within the cell; they have thick walls that can remain dormant and then be released, and they are quite resistant to infection control procedures.

Basic structure and functions of each component

Bacteria have a nucleus or nucleoid structure composed of DNA, which controls cellular activities; there may also be small plasmids containing DNA. Bacteria have a larger cytoplasm surrounding the nucleoid enclosed within a cytoplasmic membrane. The cytoplasm is relatively viscous and also contains essential macromolecules, water, oxygen, waste products, and storage granules. The surrounding cytoplasm membrane is made up of lipids and proteins and serves to regulate the transport of nutrients, metabolic functions, waste expulsion, cell wall synthesis, and DNA synthesis during cell division. Some, primarily gram-positive, bacteria have infoldings from the cytoplasm membrane into the cytoplasm containing hydrolytic enzymes. External to the cytoplasmic membrane is a rigid cell wall composed of peptidoglycan, polymers peptides and polysaccharides, which function to retain cell shape and protect to the cell from mechanical injury.

Oxygen requirement

Different types of bacteria have varying oxygen requirements. They fall into 4 categories. In 3 of these categories, the bacteria possess enzymes called superoxide dismutase (SOD) and catalase. SOD breaks down toxic superoxides into molecular oxygen and hydrogen peroxide and catalase converts the hydrogen peroxide into water and molecular oxygen. Thus, all three of these groups can thrive to a certain extent in the presence of oxygen. They are (1) obligate aerobes, which can only grow in the presence of about 20% oxygen, (2) microaerophiles, which can endure only lower concentrations of oxygen of about 4%, and (3) facultative anaerobes, which can tolerate oxygen but do not require it. The last category (4) is obligate anaerobes, which do not have SOD or catalase and cannot proliferate in the presence of oxygen.

Growth pattern

Bacterial cells divide by binary fission producing two daughter cells. Under the right conditions this fission process occurs very rapidly (minutes) through successive generations. Bacterial growth is influenced by the temperature of the environment, its acidity, the available nutrients, whether or not its oxygen requirements are met, and presence of water. Each bacterium has an optimal temperature range. Some are thermophiles, which thrive at 56°C (range 45-70°C). Most bacteria that endure in the human body fall into the second category of mesophiles, which survive at 22-45°C (optimally 37°C), and there are some bacteria that are psychrophiles, which thrive best at 1-22°C (best 7°C). Bacteria usually grow best in the human body at neutral pH 7 or in the slightly acidic to slightly alkaline range of pH 5.5 to 8.5. However, some can endure lower pHs and are known as aciduric while others generate acids during growth (acidogenic), contributing to dental decay. Bacteria have varying needs in terms of nutrients and metabolism as the presence or absence of oxygen (both discussed further on other cards).

Nutrients required and metabolic activities of bacterial cells

Metabolism in living organisms is the totality of chemical reactions within them. Nutrients must be brought into the organism and converted into the macromolecules required for sustenance. Metabolism consists of both catabolism, the breakdown of nutrients into utilizable forms, and anabolism, the synthesis of new molecules. In bacteria, nutrients enter the cell through the cytoplasmic membrane and are catabolized to generate the building blocks and energy needed for anabolism. Catabolism can occur through fermentation or respiration. Fermentation is the anaerobic splitting of sugars, ultimately producing lactic acid that contributes to caries formation. Respiration occurs aerobically. Here sugars are broken down into pyruvic acid, which undergoes a course called the electron transport chain and generates ATP. ATP, adenosine triphosphate, is an energy source for synthesis during anabolism. Both respiration and fermentation generate waste products. Metabolic processes require enzymes or protein catalysts and sometimes metallic cofactors or organic coenzymes. Anabolic processes generate needed proteins, nucleic acids, lipids, polysaccharides, and vitamins within the bacterial cell.

Ways bacteria are cultured in laboratory

In the laboratory, bacteria are cultured either in a liquid broth or on a semi-solid agar medium made up of a polysaccharide derived from seaweed. Both are sterilized by boiling and are then cooled before use, and particular nutrients are added. Using sterile technique, potential bacterial cultures are inoculated into broth cultures to observe for turbidity or opaqueness indicating growth. Likewise, they are streaked onto plates containing the agar medium, which separates them into cells or groups thereof called colony-forming units (CFUs). Subsequent plates can be streaked further with individual CFUs to obtain pure clones or colonies. Specific bacteria have characteristic growth media (containing set nutrients or incubated under certain conditions) in which they thrive and proliferate, thus, aiding in identification.

Regulating growth

Bacterial growth can be prevented, and bacteria can be killed. Agents or states that can thwart bacterial growth but not actually kill bacteria are referred to as bacteriostatic. Bacteriostatic measures include freezing to shatter the cell membrane, refrigeration (unless the bacteria thrive at that temperature), regulating oxygen levels (depending on the type of suspected bacteria), or use of extreme pH. Situations that kill bacteria are termed bactericidal. The most effective bactericidal measure is exposure to extremely high temperatures through steam, dry heat, or chemical vapor sterilizers, which can break down bacterial proteins, nucleic acids, and structures. There are chemicals that can kill bacteria on inert objects (such as surfaces) and are therefore bactericidal.

Similar destruction of viruses or fungi is termed virucidal or fungicidal respectively. In the body, bacteria can be inhibited or in some cases killed by use of antibiotics.

Properties that make microorganisms pathogenic

Depending on the specific microorganism, a microorganism may have properties that enhance infection, interfere with host defenses, and/or directly damage cells or tissues. Infection enhancement properties include means of attachment to host cells (for example fimbriae or surface polymers on certain bacteria and through the capsid or envelope on viruses) and ability to multiply at a body site by utilizing nutrients. One additional dental application is the resistance of *Lactobacillus acidophilus* to acids. There are many ways in which microorganisms interfere with host defenses. These include things such as destruction of phagocytes, inhibition of their attraction by certain extracellular products, ways to evade engulfment or digestion by phagocytes, or mechanisms that suppress or circumvent the immune system. The latter is particularly true for viruses such as HIV, herpes simplex, and influenza. The last category of properties includes microorganisms that damage cells or tissues. There are numerous microorganisms in this category. Certain bacteria produce histolytic enzymes, serotoxins, cytotoxic waste products, and endotoxins or persist in chronic forms that eventually damage the immune system. The latter is also true for certain viruses.

Microbiology of dental caries

Dental caries or decay starts when acidogenic or acid-producing bacteria on the teeth are present in an environment of a susceptible host and sugars in the diet. The dietary sugars are metabolized producing acids, which accumulate at the tooth surface to create a low pH acidic environment leading to demineralization or loss of tooth structure. After demineralization (indicated by white spots on the teeth) dental caries or tooth decay will result. Decay development only occurs if there is a susceptible host, presence of caries-causing bacteria in the form of dental plaque or impactions, the correct substrate (sucrose or other sugars), and time for development. Plaque is actually a biofilm of bacteria entrenched in an intercellular matrix of other molecules, particularly glycoproteins from saliva, that coat the tooth surface with a thin layer called the pellicle.

Normal oral microbiota

Newborns acquire microorganisms during passage through the mother's birth canal, but most of these do not remain as normal oral microbiota. During childhood, kids are exposed to environmental organisms that become part of their oral microbiota if they affix to oral surfaces and multiply. When new teeth erupt, microorganisms can also enter the oral cavity through bleeding. By the early teens, the normal oral flora is generally established as a mixture of as many as 40 types of bacteria genera and often the yeast *Candida albicans*. Saliva and plaque contain millions of bacteria.

Plaque-associated periodontal diseases

Periodontal diseases at the neck or root of a tooth develop because plaque-associated bacteria and their harmful products accrue in these areas causing tissue damage, inflammation, and immune interactions. When plaque is allowed to accumulate, the bacteria in it produce potentially harmful products, such as endotoxins and serotoxins, noxious metabolites, histolytic enzymes, and substances with immune effects, such as antigens, immunosuppressants, and antiphagocytic factors. These cause damage to the periodontal tissues and elicit immune responses. The result can be simple gingivitis, which is inflammation and possibly bleeding that can be reversed with plaque removal. It can also be necrotizing ulcerative gingivitis or trench mouth, which is also reversible. If, however, there are inaccessible bacteria-filled periodontal pockets, periodontitis is the diagnosis. This can lead to chronic periodontitis in which bone is slowly and progressively destroyed or in people with weak body defenses, other forms of periodontitis. Many gram-negative bacteria are found in subgingival plaque as opposed to the most prevalent caries-causing bacteria, which are gram-positive.

Bacteria likely to cause caries

The bacteria present that are most likely to cause caries are mutans streptococci (*Streptococcus mutans or Streptococcus sobrinus*), which are acidogenic, aciduric, and tend to build up on the teeth. Mutans streptococci have enzymes called glucosyltransferases that break down sucrose into polysaccharide glucans and bind to cells encouraging further plaque formation and fructose which is ultimately processed into lactic acid. *Lactobacillus* species are also conducive to caries formation as they are acidogenic and acid uric, but they do not have good ways to attach to tooth surfaces by themselves. *Actinomyces naeslundii* if present are conducive to plaque formation and in particular development of root caries.

Acute dental and other oral infections

Pulpitis, which is inflammation of the pulp of the tooth, is caused when caries spreads into the pulp region. Pulpitis can spread further to the apex or periapical region and in some cases to the adjacent facial tissues as cellulitis or inflammation of subcutaneous tissues. Pulpitis is generally treated endodontically by a root canal procedure, which is the removal of dead pulp tissue, killing and pulling out bacteria in the root canal and adding inert materials to the canals. Antibiotics may also be given. Transient bacteremia, in which normal oral microbiota get into the bloodstream because of oral bleeding, can be a problem. Individuals with heart valve damage, for example, can experience further injury or subacute bacterial endocarditis (inflammation of the heart). Rarely *Actinomyces* species can cause jaw, neck, or lung infections.

Generalizations about viruses

Viruses are very small (0.3 microns or less) microorganisms consisting of a central nucleic acid core (either DNA or RNA) and a protein coat called the capsid. Certain viruses also have an external envelope made of proteins, polysaccharides, and lipids. Viruses cannot replicate unless they exist within a susceptible host such as the human body. Their life cycle is initiated by adsorption or attachment to the host cell. This is followed by penetration of the host cell, uncoating of the capsid (which discharges the viral nucleic acid), replication (which is use of the host cell to generate new viral nucleic acid and capsid), assembly of a new viral particle, and release of it upon lysis of the host cell (enabling the virus to infect other cells). If the viral nucleic acid remains integrated into the host DNA, it continues to be replicated, lying latent or dormant until some later event reactivates the virus. Viruses can also cause chronic or slow persistent infections. Certain viruses transform host cells but do not lyse them, often resulting in tumors. Viruses can be killed on surfaces with measures used for bacteria, but they cannot be killed inside the body.

Infections caused by rickettsiae

Rickettsiae are tiny parasitic microorganisms that live in and multiply in a variety of hosts. These microorganisms are transmitted by the host to humans. The transporter is usually a flea or tick, which in some cases, is carried by a rodent. In terms of dentistry, the rickettsiae of greatest interest are those spread by head lice to school age children, causing pediculosis. Head lice are small, bloodsucking, wingless parasites that produce eggs that can be visualized on hair shafts. Measures such as medicinal shampoos, combing, and hot water washing of all clothing and bedding are needed to rid the child of these microorganisms. Most other rickettsial diseases are rare, including Rocky Mountain Spotted Fever, which causes flulike symptoms and pick spotting, and typhus, which rapidly causes high fever, headache, pain in the back and extremities, confusion, a rash, and weakening of the heart beat.

Infections caused by protozoa

Protozoa or amoebas are single-celled microorganisms. They are often found in contaminated water and can survive in bodily fluids such as blood or in the fluid found in the oral cavity or intestinal tract. They are larger than bacteria (about 100 microns) and reproduce by binary fission. They entrap food in a unique manner by altering their shape to surround and ingest food and incorporate it into an internal food vacuole. These shape changes also help with mobility as do the flagella possessed by many of these organisms. Protozoa are important in dentistry for several reasons. They usually contribute to periodontal disease along with bacteria by their presence in periodontal pockets. One important protozoal disease is amebic dysentery, which is caused by *Entamoeba histolytica* and is characterized by serious diarrhea and occasionally liver abscesses. Protozoa are also responsible for malaria and sleeping sickness spread via mosquito and tsetse fly bites respectively in tropical countries.

Infections caused by fungi

Fungi are generally spore-producing microorganisms that reproduce by budding. They may be single- or multicellular. They lack chlorophyll, making them nonphotosynthetic, and they are eukaryotic with visible nuclei and organelles. Molds and yeast are forms of fungi causing infections. Mushrooms also are considered fungi. The fungus of greatest interest is *Candida albicans*, which causes candidiasis (also known as thrush or moniliasis). *C. albicans* is a constituent of many individual's normal flora, but it is an opportunistic infection that can take over when a person's immune defenses are lowered such as in presence of AIDS or overuse of antibiotics. Thrush is characterized by raised white or cream-colored patches in the oral cavity. It can be painful and should be treated with antifungal drugs. Tinea is a group of fungal infections. Variants are tinea pedis or athlete's foot, tinea corporus or ringworm, and tinea unguium, which are white patches on nails. Oral and/or topical fungal medications are indicated.

Endogenous and exogenous infectious diseases

Infectious diseases are illnesses caused by multiplication of harmful microorganisms or pathogens in the body and subsequent tissue damage. They can be classified as endogenous or exogenous depending on the source of the infection. Endogenous infectious diseases are produced by microorganisms generally present on or in the body without untoward effect. These microorganisms can be opportunistic, however, and if certain events occur they can take over or penetrate areas and become harmful. In the dental setting, normal oral flora can cause endogenous diseases such as decay, periodontal disease, and pulpitis. Exogenous infectious diseases are ones that are caused by microorganisms not generally present invading the body. Most infectious diseases fall into this category. These external exogenous microbes can act directly by penetrating the body and multiplying or they can produce toxins or poisons with untoward effects (known as toxigenic diseases).

Oral diseases

Viral origin

Oral diseases of viral origin are primarily caused by some type of human herpesvirus or coxsackievirus. There are 8 types of DNA-containing human herpes viruses (HHV-1 to -8). Oral lesions known as cold sores or aphthous ulcers are primarily caused by HHV-1, occasionally by the predominantly genital type HHV-2 (also known as herpes simplex types 1 and 2), and as infectious mononucleosis or hairy leukoplakia of the tongue by HHV-4 (Epstein-Barr virus). Herpesviruses trigger recurrent episodes because they are retained on nerve ganglia and can be reactivated. Direct contact with anyone having active lesions such as fever blisters or herpes labialis can result in transmission. In the dental setting, a healthcare worker touching a lesion directly can get herpetic willow on his or her hands. There is also some possibility of contracting the virus even if the patient is asymptomatic. Coxsackievirus can cause herpangina, vesicles generally found in the back of the mouth, or hand-foot-and-mouth disease in which there are vesicles on many oral areas such as the cheek and tongue.

Bacterial or fungal origin

Pharyngitis, inflammation of the pharynx, can be caused by two main types of bacteria: *Neisseria gonorrhoeae* and Streptococcus *pyogenes*. *N. gonorrhoeae* is primarily sexually transmitted but can be found orally after engaging in certain practices. *Streptococcus pyogenes,* technically a respiratory disease, causes strep throat or scarlet fever as well as skin infections and is carried by up to 20% of children. *Streptococcus mutans* is another species linked to dental caries and endocarditis. The other bacterial disease with oral manifestations is syphilis, caused by the spirochete *Treponema pallidum.* Normally syphilis is a systemic disease but oral lesions or chancres containing the spirochete can be found in up to 10% of instances. The main fungus causing oral manifestations is the opportunistic yeast *Candida albicans*. It proliferates under certain opportune conditions such as depression of the immune system with HIV or leukemia, lengthy use of broad-spectrum antibiotics, mouth trauma usually from poorly fitting dentures, or transmission during birth. The possible oral manifestations are candidiasis or thrush, which are whitish lesions, and denture stomatitis, which appears as reddish regions.

Hepatitis B virus

Viral hepatitis caused by hepatitis B virus

Hepatitis B virus (HBV) is one form of viral hepatitis, which is inflammation of the liver. HBV is a double-stranded DNA hepadnavirus. It is a bloodborne disease, meaning it is transmitted via blood or bodily fluids; it has been found to be spread parenterally, sexually, through skin or mucous membrane contact, perinatally, through sharing of contaminated needles by intravenous drug users, and through other fluid contact. HBV is rarely spread through transfusions these days because of the excellent blood screening tests now available. After an incubation period of about 45-180 days after exposure, hepatitis symptoms usually show up gradually. About two-thirds of those exposed are asymptomatic or have mild symptoms; less than 1% have fulminant or severe hepatitis, and the rest become symptomatic (jaundice, dark urine, joint pain, fever, etc). Most people exposed to HBV recover, but about 5 to 10% become carriers (hepatitis B surface antigen positive). About half of these individuals clear the infection within 5 years but the other half become chronic carriers of the virus, predisposing them to hepatocellular carcinoma and cirrhosis, progressive liver disease.

Risk of transmission in dental setting

Dental workers who are not vaccinated against B virus are at least twice as likely as the general public to contract hepatitis B virus. Over the last few decades, this risk has been cut down tremendously because several vaccines that provide protection against HBV have been developed. OSHA, the Occupational and Safety and Health Administration, now requires all health care professions, including dental offices, to offer HBV vaccines free of charge to anyone with potential bloodborne exposure. Those who take the vaccines and show seroconversion are protected against the virus. The biggest occupational threats for infection with HBV are punctures with contaminated sharps, exposure to blood or saliva through skin cuts or cracks, or spraying of these fluids into lacerations or mucous membranes. Since dentists and other dental personnel are usually vaccinated, the risk of dental worker to patient transmission is minimal. There is possibility of patient-to-patient spread of the virus. HBV can be viable for a month or more at room temperature, but general office sterilization and disinfection procedures should kill the virus.

Important antigens and antibodies

The most important antigen is HBsAg, hepatitis B surface antigen. HBsAg is a soluble antigen detectable in serum during periods of active infection or in the carrier state for hepatitis B. Antibody to HBsAg, anti-HBs, is indicative, when found in the serum, of past HBV infection and development of immunity through exposure, vaccination, or passive administration of HBIG (hepatitis B immune globulin). The other important HBV antigens are the hepatitis B core antigen (HBcAg) and hepatitis B e antigen (HBeAg) proteins. HBeAg, which is closely related to HBcAg, is soluble and correlates with evidence of HBV replication; thus, it is indicative of current HBV infection when found in serum. Appearance of its antibody, anti-HBe, implies a lowering of viral titer. There are also tests for antibodies to the core protein, anti-HBc and IgM anti-HBc, which if present, point to prior or recent infection with HBV respectively. Presence of antibodies to both surface and core antigens signify immunity. The actual HBV virus or Dane particle can also be looked for, although this is not routinely done.

Hepatitis C virus infection

Hepatitis B, C and D viruses are bloodborne. Hepatitis C virus (HCV) is an enveloped single-stranded RNA flavivirus. Its incubation period is from one to five months and its onset is usually insidious. The routes of transmission are similar to those for HBV except that about half of cases have been found to be related to intravenous drug abuse. Unlike HBV, most (up to 85%) of HCV-infected individuals go on to be chronic carriers of the virus and about 1/5 of those contract chronic liver disease including hepatocellular carcinoma and cirrhosis. There is no current vaccine. There is a risk of contracting the virus in the dental setting, although it is less than for HBV transmission because the virus is less virulent. There are good available screening tests for anti-HCV, antibody to HCV. Presence of anti-HCV indicates current or previous HCV infection, although it does not pinpoint the acute, chronic, or resolved state.

Hepatitis D infection

Hepatitis D virus (HDV) is a bloodborne, non-enveloped, single-stranded RNA virus. It only exists as a satellite or defective virus; in other words, it is only capable of infection in the presence of hepatitis B virus. It is spread like other bloodborne pathogens. The incubation period is from 21 to 90 days and symptoms are generally acute. The primary antigen of HDV is Delta antigen or Hdag. It is demonstrable in early acute delta infection, and its antibody, anti-HDV, if found indicates current or past infection. HDV can exist chronically in carrier states and cause hepatocellular carcinoma and cirrhosis. Acute infection with HDV, which can only occur in conjunction with HBV coinfection, can result in death in up to 30% of cases. If antibody to hepatitis B surface antigen (anti-HBsAg) is detectable in the serum, an individual is immune to HDV as well. Because the virus is bloodborne, it presents an occupational hazard in the dental setting.

HIV infection

Course of infection

Human immunodeficiency viruses 1 and 2 (HIV-1 and HIV-2) are single-stranded RNA retroviruses. HIV-1 is more common, particularly in the United States. A retrovirus replicates within a host cell, in this case primarily helper T4 or CD4 lymphocytes, by using its RNA as a template to make viral DNA copies, which are integrated into the chromosomes of the host's lymphocytes. This leads to formation of viral particles within and destruction and depletion of T4 lymphocytes. Within about a month after infection with HIV, a person may exhibit mild symptoms such as fever, enlarged glands, or fatigue. These symptoms comprise acute retroviral syndrome. The individual will develop anti-HIV antibodies and seroconvert within the next few weeks to months, but these antibodies are not protective and replication and T4 lymphocyte killing continues. The individual usually appears relatively asymptomatic until his or her immune system has become undermined enough to generate the symptoms of AIDS (acquired immunodeficiency syndrome). These symptoms include susceptibility to opportunistic infections such fungal pneumonia from *Pneumocystis jiroveci* or malignancies, including rare ones such as Kaposi's sarcoma.

Dental manifestations of HIV infection and risk of transmission

Once an individual reaches the early stages of acquired immunodeficiency syndrome (AIDS), many of the first indications are oral, including candidiasis or thrush, histoplasmosis, warts, periodontitis or gingivitis from bacterial infections, Kaposi's sarcoma, and others. The documented and potential transmission to dental workers is much lower than for some other types of healthcare workers such as nurses or laboratory personnel. Nevertheless, any healthcare worker who incurs some type of puncture or cut and is exposed to HIV-positive blood has the greatest chance of contracting the virus. To date, there has only been one dentist implicated in transmission of HIV to patients. Common dental practices using personal protective equipment, disinfection, and sterilization virtually eliminate patient exposure to the virus. For example, HIV is readily deactivated with heat or gas sterilization and by most liquid sterilizers and surface disinfectants. In addition, contaminated sharps must be dealt with carefully and disposed of properly to reduce potential exposure.

Tuberculosis

Tuberculosis and possibility of transmission

One of the biggest concerns globally is the possibility of contraction of tuberculosis, a respiratory infection caused by *Mycobacterium tuberculosis*. Persons at greatest risk for contraction of tuberculosis are those in intimate and prolonged contact with an active carrier or individuals who have a compromised immune system. The symptoms of tuberculosis are a lengthy productive cough, blood in the sputum, headache, fever and night sweats, loss of weight, and a general weariness. Since tuberculosis is transmitted by prolonged exposure to concentrated amounts of the bacteria in airborne droplets, the risk of spread in a dental office is low but possible. Generally, dental work should not be done on individuals with active tuberculosis. Active disease is characterized by pneumonia or another exudative lung condition, formation of tubercles or fusion of granulomatous tissues if more advanced, and eventually lung tissue destruction. There may also be complications in other organs where the bacteria have traveled via macrophages. Drugs used to treat tuberculosis include rifampin, isoniazid, and ethambutol, but many strains are resistant to one or more agents.

Amount of induration on a tuberculin skin test

Individuals with positive skin tests are considered recent converters if the size of induration becomes more intense over a two year period. The cutoffs are increases of at least 10 mm if the person is younger than 35 and at least 15 mm if they are 35 years of age or older. Dental and other healthcare workers should be subject to the same recommendations for interpretation of the skin test as others (described elsewhere). Healthcare workers should be considered recently exposed to tuberculosis if the 2 year increase in induration is greater than or equal to 10 mm, although the 15 mm cutoff is sometimes used.

Interpretation of tuberculin skin test

The tuberculin skin test, also known as the Mantoux test or purified protein derivative (PPD) test, is a screening check for exposure to *Mycobacterium tuberculosis*. A small quantity of PPD is injected intradermally on the underside of the forearm. The test is usually read 2 to 3 days later. The amount of induration or hardening of the injected is noted, keeping in mind various factors. In general, anyone with an induration of $\geq$ 15 mm is considered positive. Smaller indurations of $\geq$ 5 mm are deemed positive in individuals with HIV or risk factors for the disease, those who have been in recent contact with people with active tuberculosis, or those who have fibrotic chest radiographs consistent with healed disease. The cutoff is $\geq$ 10 mm for the following high-risk groups: HIV-negative IV drug users; those with medical conditions that could be complicated by active TB, such as bypass, renal failure, diabetes, or hematologic disease patients; young children; other high-prevalence groups, such as people born outside the United States and Europe; those in low-income groups; and people in long-term care facilities.

CDC guidelines for preventing tuberculosis in dental settings

The CDC (Centers for Disease Control) recommends that infection control in a dental setting be based on regular risk assessment for *Mycobacterium tuberculosis* exposure, usually using PPD skin testing. Infection control should include evaluation of tuberculosis in the community and in the dental office. There is minimal risk of exposure if none were reported in either setting or very low risk if none were seen in the office. There is low probability if fewer than 6 patients with active disease were seen the previous year and no dental workers seroconverted. If more patients had active tuberculosis or dental workers seroconvert, the risk is intermediate or high respectively. Routine practices should also include documentation of tuberculosis in the patient's history, referral for assessment of those patients with potential tuberculosis (based on history or signs), provision of surgical masks to these patients, delay of elective procedures until full evaluation, isolation of patients requiring critical care if tuberculosis is suspected, evaluation and temporary removal of dental workers presenting with tuberculosis-type symptoms (such as persistent cough for at least 3 weeks), and provision of state of the art engineering if tuberculosis patients are treated.

Emerging diseases

Emerging diseases are previously unrecognized new infectious diseases. Many of these emerging diseases evolve through close contact with animal (zoonotic) contacts or insect vectors. Rodents are common animal vectors and mosquitoes and ticks are frequent insect vectors. Over the last few decades, an average of one emerging disease per year has been identified with the majority being viral. Changing demographics, such as movement into cities, overcrowding, and the increase in international travel and business dealings, account for some of these discoveries. Technological advances, while beneficial, can encourage transmission of infectious agents to new areas, for example by global food distribution methods or water-handling devices. Many microorganisms can mutate into slightly-modified new forms. The best examples are the constantly changing influenza virus and antibiotic-resistant forms of various bacteria.

Dental Water

Microorganisms found in dental unit water

General water is supplied to a dental office by municipal facilities. At the point of origin, the water is non-sterile but low in microbial growth, typically from 0 to 500 CFU/mL. CFU stands for a colony-forming unit, a single or small number of bacteria that can develop further. The same water that is supplied to the rest of the office (faucets, etc.) is also delivered to the dental unit except that the hoses for the latter are narrower inviting microbial growth. Typical dental unit water in untreated systems contains over 100,000 CFU/mL and often much higher levels of microbial growth. Numerous species of bacteria derived from both the water and patient's mouths have been identified in dental unit water. Some of these bacteria are opportunistic and pathogenic. A number of species of fungi and protozoa have also been recognized in dental water, but those identified have low pathogenicity.

The microorganisms found in dental water of most concern are various species of *Pseudomonas, Legionella pneumophila,* and nontuberculous species of *Mycobacterium. Pseudomonas* species often thrive in the water supply and are opportunistic and pathogenic. Two in particular are of concern, *P. aeruginosa,* which can cause urinary tract and wound infection, pneumonia, and possibly septicemia and *P. cepacia,* which causes respiratory problems in patients with cystic fibrosis. *Legionella pneumophila* (as well as other species) is a water-borne bacterium that can cause respiratory issues and to a lesser extent wound infections and Pontiac fever. Other opportunistic pathogens have been identified in dental water units in addition to those mentioned. In addition, studies suggest that the levels of endotoxins, toxic substances released from the cell walls of dead gram-negative bacteria, can be higher than desirable.

Biofilm

Biofilm is a mass or layer of microorganisms directly attached to a surface with moisture exposure. There are numerous types of biofilm in nature, but the ones of interest in dentistry are dental plaque and biofilm attached to the interior of a dental unit water line. In a water line some bacterial growth is free-floating or planktonic. Those bacteria that affix to a surface, in this case the internal walls of the water line, form cell surface polymers called exopolysaccharides or glycocalyx polymers, which enlarge as new bacterial cells are recruited from the planktonic portion forming a slimy surface biofilm.

A number of factors contribute to formation of dental unit water line biofilm. Water within the tubing stagnates when the unit is not being used. The tubing feeding the unit is small in diameter which means there is a large surface to volume ratio facilitating bacterial contact and attachment to the surface. Many of these waterborne bacteria have characteristics that encourage surface attachment. They are always present in some concentration, and as they attach to the walls of the line they multiply, increasing the biofilm mass. In addition, other bacteria can enter the dental unit water line from the air, at water line openings, or through retraction through the handpiece or air/water syringe. Water surging past the attached biofilm can acquire bacteria from the biofilm passing it into the handpiece, air/water syringe, and other equipment.

Dental unit water quality

Monitoring
If measures are being taken to improve the quality of dental unit water, their effectiveness should be monitored at baseline and at regular intervals. Water samples are taken and either shipped cold

to a facility for testing (such as a microbiology laboratory or dental company) or tested in-house. The testing involves neutralizing the water sample in diluted chlorine, inoculating it onto a specific type of agar plate called R2A and then incubating the plate at room temperature for a minimum of a week before determining bacterial counts. Dental unit water quality measures are considered effective if the bacterial counts are less than 500 colony-forming units (CFU)/mL. However, this testing is only approximate because the relationship between amount of biofilm on the water line and the concentration of bacteria in a particular water sample has not been established.

Improving

One approach is to disconnect from the municipal water supply and set up an independent water reservoir for delivery of dental treatment water. This is discussed further on another card. Another tactic is to use decontaminating and antimicrobial agents in independent water reservoirs. Depending on the agent, they can be flushed periodically thru the water lines or put directly into the treatment water. Municipal water systems use other means of destroying microorganisms such as ultraviolet light or heating. Placing an antimicrobial filter in the line just ahead of where the water enters the handpiece or air/water syringe can filter out free-floating microorganisms and in some instances endotoxin. Filters must be changed regularly. All devices used must be FDA-cleared, and all chemicals utilized must be registered by the EPA. FDA-approved sterile water delivery systems, which completely circumvent the dental unit lines, should be used for surgical procedures.

Boil water notice

A boil water notice is a warning issued by authorities to boil municipal water before using it for drinking, bathing, or healthcare-related activities. Boil water notices are released by the water company or health officials because some type of problem has occurred in the municipal water treatment plant or water distribution system. Implications of an issued boil water notice in the dental office are that municipal water should not be used for any sort of patient treatment or handwashing. Offices that use an independent water reservoir for the dental unit can still treat patients but must find some other means of handwashing. If they normally use municipal water for the dental unit, syringe irrigation with other water (for example distilled) must be used or patient care must be suspended. Once the boil water notice has been lifted, the dental water lines must be disinfected and flushed per manufacturer's or local authority's instructions or if unknown for 5 minutes before use.

Using an independent water reservoir for dental unit

Use of an independent water reservoir to deliver treatment water, circumventing the municipal water system, is one way of improving the quality of dental unit water. The unit is disconnected from the municipal water system and the independent water reservoir is attached instead for water delivery. Initially on three consecutive evenings cleaner/disinfectant is added to a bottle, the bottle is connected to the dental water line and pressurized to flush the cleaner through the system, and is left that way overnight. The subsequent morning the bottle is taken off, the pickup line rinsed, and another bottle with water is connected and run through the same type of flushing. After three sets of cleaner then water flushing, a clean bottle with distilled water is connected to the unit and pressurized for use. Distilled water has been boiled to reduce microbial counts. After each patient day, the water reservoir with distilled water is emptied and put back on the unit and pressurized to blow out excess water. The next morning, a clean bottle with distilled treatment water is attached and pressurized for use. Once a week, flushing with cleaner/disinfectant (as described above) is done once before connecting a new treatment bottle.

Bacteria of concern that can be transmitted via dental unit water

Dental units and hoses harbor waterborne bacteria and viruses. Some of the bacteria affix to the inside of the water lines forming a biofilm, which can then be discharged upon use. While as many as 40 species of bacteria might be present, the two of most concern are *Legionella pneumophila* and *Pseudomonas aeruginosa*. *L. pneumophila* causes Legionnaires' disease (lung infections characterized by pneumonia) through inhalation of contaminated water or drawing in of bacteria already colonizing the oropharyngeal region. The agent can also produce the flu-like Pontiac fever. The other waterborne bacterium of interest is *P. aeruginosa*, which can generate oral infections in susceptible individuals. Dental units also may have low levels of oral bacteria in their water supply due to retraction. The CDC and the ADA suggest that dental unit water should not be employed for irrigation of exposed surgical sites and that lines should be rinsed out first thing in the morning and between patients.

The Body's Defense System

Natural host defense barriers to infection

There are 4 types of natural or innate host defense barriers to infection. There are physical barriers such as intact skin and mucous membranes at various sites (mouth, eyes, respiratory tree, etc.). There are also mechanical barriers to infection that cleanse the system of the microorganisms. These include oral saliva and mucus, a cilia escalator that traps and moves inhaled particles back out the mouth, the regular shedding of skin and mucous membrane cells, nasal hair, and expulsion through coughing or sneezing. The body produces a number of chemicals with antimicrobial properties, such as hydrochloric acid in the stomach, organic acids on the skin and vaginal area, lysozyme in the saliva and other secretions, a whole complex of components called the complement system, and the mainly antiviral substance called interferon. Lastly, the white blood cells neutrophils and macrophages act as phagocytes to surround and destroy microorganisms.

Protective actions of antibodies

Antibodies bind to foreign antigens, such as those on microorganisms, present in the body. Through their binding properties, they can augment phagocytic destruction of microorganisms either directly or through activation of the complement system. Antibodies can deter attachment of the agent to host cells; they might inactivate toxins or histolytic enzymes by binding to certain destructive molecules; they can lyse gram-negative bacteria or enveloped viruses through activation of the complement system, and they can also lyse virus-infected cells by binding to both those cells and macrophages. The main goal of vaccination or immunization is the injection of antigens that have been modified enough so that they won't cause harmful effects but will generate protective antibodies. It is hoped that vaccination or immunization will create long-term, artificially-created immunity. Protective antibodies are of the IgG class, or early in infection, the IgM class.

Acquired defenses that fight infections

When a microorganism invades the human body, immune responses are activated to prevent harmful damage and impart protection against further assault with the same agent. The immune responses are mounted against antigens or substances that the body considers foreign, generally specific portions of the infectious agent. Certain macrophages process these antigens via phagocytes; they interact with T and B lymphocytes, which clonally expand and recognize the antigens, and responses are generated against the invading agent. These responses are of two types. Cell-mediated responses involve activated T lymphocytes, which can act in several ways by either controlling antibody-mediated responses, obliterating infected cells, generating chemicals called lymphokines that activate other cells like phagocytes, or destroying modified host cells (such as malignant ones). There are also antibody-mediated responses in which protein antibodies specifically recognizing and binding to foreign antigens are created utilizing B lymphocytes.

Harmful immune responses

The main way in which the immune system causes harmful responses is through development of allergic diseases. Allergic manifestations can occur in the nose or eyes (hay fever), the respiratory tract (asthma), as skin rashes (hives), or systemically as anaphylactic shock. Most of these reactions are to pollens and other environmental allergens such as pet dander or to foods. Both antibody-mediated responses (elicited by a class of antibody called IgE) and cell-mediated responses to antigens (allergens) can occur. Certain chronic infections can also precipitate cell-mediated allergic responses. Contact dermatitis is a form of cell-mediated allergic reaction to certain chemicals such as the oils from poison ivy, nickel in jewelry, or latex. Allergic responses are generally evaluated by doing skin tests, and there are also immunoassays available measuring IgE in serum. Individuals may overcome their allergies if they develop enough of what are called blocking antibodies to the offending antigen.

Immunizations

Influenza infections

Influenza respiratory infections are characterized clinically by acute onset, high fever (up to 104°F), severe headache and other pains, prolonged fatigue, and cough and severe chest discomfort in most cases. Stuffy nose, sneezing, and sore throat are more characteristic of colds, not the flu. Influenza can lead to critical complications such as bronchitis, pneumonia, and even death. The incubation period for the virus is 1 to 4 days and virus is maximally shed around the onset of symptoms. The mode of transmission is generally aerosols or droplets, although direct contact is sometimes implicated. There are two types of influenza, types A and B, and variants within those two types. The CDC suggests annual single-dose vaccination with preparations prepared each year to reflect the expected culprits in the hemisphere where administered. There are two kinds of vaccine, an inactivated or killed vaccine that is administered intramuscularly, and a live, attenuated or weakened vaccine (LAIV) given intranasally. The intramuscular, inactivated form is recommended for most people including healthcare workers. LAIV should only be given to non-pregnant individuals ages 5 to 49. There are antiviral medications available, but these are not realistic options.

Contraindications for influenza vaccines

All influenza vaccines are currently prepared using eggs. Therefore, people allergic to eggs or other constituents of the vaccine should not receive it as they may develop critical anaphylactic hypersensitivity reactions. There are a number of contraindications for the LAIV vaccine as it contains live, albeit weakened, influenza virus and is given in a form (intranasally) quickly accessible to the respiratory tract. Only healthy, nonpregnant individuals between the ages of 5 and 49 should take this vaccine. People outside these age ranges, those with chronic pulmonary or cardiovascular diseases, anyone with underlying medical conditions like diabetes or renal disease, people with known or possible immunodeficiency diseases, those with Guillain-Barré syndrome, and pregnant women should not take the live attenuated influenza vaccine. Children or adolescents who are taking aspirin or calculates should not take the LAIV vaccine either because of its association with the childhood disease called Reye syndrome, but they should receive the inactivated influenza vaccine. Individuals in intimate contact with immunosuppressed patients, for example certain healthcare workers, should also refrain from receiving the LAIV vaccine.

Immunization of dental health care personnel

Hepatitis B

Hepatitis B virus (HBV) presents a significant occupational hazard for dental health care personnel (DHCP) if they are not vaccinated. The bloodborne virus is quite virulent and stable. It causes both acute and chronic symptoms, including liver cirrhosis, necrotizing vasculitis, and hepatocellular carcinoma. OSHA requirements regarding immunization are discussed elsewhere. Some version of the recombinant Hepatitis B vaccine is recommended for DHCP and other at risk adults. The administration schedule is 2 doses 4 weeks apart given intramuscularly in the deltoid muscle followed by a third dose 5 months later. The available single antigen vaccines are Recombivax HB and Energix-B, and there are combination vaccines containing HBV antigens along with others (Twinrix for adults, Comvax and Pediarix for children). Serologic tests for anti-HBsAg to measure protective effects should be done one to two months after completion of the dose series. Individuals who are exposed to HBV but are not immune should be given hepatitis B immune globulin, 0.6 mL/kg intramuscularly within 7 days of exposure. This should be followed by another round a month later if the HBV vaccine series has not been initiated.

New employees should be offered the hepatitis B vaccination series (generally 3 spaced injections) within 10 days of employment and after receiving training. The vaccine should be offered free of charge and administered by a licensed physician or nurse practitioner in an office where the OSHA Bloodborne Pathogens Standard is available. Potential employees need not be prescreened for hepatitis B immunity, and after employment they are not required to accept the vaccination offer. However, if they do not accept at that that time, they must sign a vaccination refusal statement. The physician must sign a written confirmation for those employees who are vaccinated. Vaccination also involves testing for effectiveness, measurement of antibody to hepatitis B surface antigen 1 to 2 months after the series. Non-responders should be advised further. There should also be an annual review of employee records to ensure that they are up-to-date on other immunizations that are deemed important.

Tetanus

Tetanus is characterized by acute hypertonia and sweeping muscles spasms, usually initially in the jaw and neck area. It is important because even though the incidence is low in the United States, tetanus remains a global problem and can cause death. Tetanus or so-called lockjaw is caused by the toxins released by the bacterium *Clostridium tetani*. Most children are given immunizations with tetanus toxoid, an inactivated form of the toxin, in conjunction with diphtheria and pertussis in a combination DPT vaccine. They are given 3 to 4 doses during the first year of life followed by boosters. The CDC recommends booster shots every 10 years into adulthood to maintain antitoxin levels or earlier if an individual has some sort of traumatic injury. The latter is suggested because *C. tetani* bacilli and spores are transmitted from environments where they flourish (such as soil) to the bloodstream through open cuts and wounds.

Varicella zoster

Varicella zoster virus (VZV or HHV-3) is responsible both for childhood chickenpox and for its adult recurrent form, shingles. The HHV-3 is retained on nerve ganglia and can reactivate in later life. Shingles is characterized by red bumps that evolve into blisters that cause inflammation and pain. It is suggested that dental health care personnel (DHCP) receive varicella zoster live virus vaccine in two 0.5 mL doses given subcutaneously given 4 to 8 weeks apart if they do not have a reliable history of previous infection or laboratory confirmation of immunity. It is cost effective to do serologic tests before vaccinating because the vast majority of people are immune. Vaccination is contraindicated in pregnant women, immunocompromised individuals, and those with history of anaphylactic reactions to gelatin or neomycin. Salicylate (aspirin) should be avoided for 6 weeks post vaccination. DHCP should also receive varicella zoster immune globulin (VZIG) if they are not immune, are susceptible to infection (for example pregnant women), and are in contact with infectious individuals. VZIG is given at a dose of 125 units/10kg up to 625 units.

Measles, mumps, and rubella

The available vaccines for measles, mumps, and rubella all contain live virus. A combined vaccine called MMR is generally the vaccine of choice if it is felt that the person is susceptible to more than one virus. All are contraindicated during pregnancy, if the person is immunocompromised, or if the individual has shown an allergic, anaphylactic reaction to gelatin, neomycin, or, in the case of measles, immune globulin. The MMR or separate vaccines are given subcutaneously in a single dose with no booster. The exception is measles vaccine, which requires a booster at least a month after the first shot. The decision of whether to receive these vaccines is somewhat dependent on age as anyone who was born before 1957 can be assumed to be immune. Nevertheless, vaccination should be considered if the worker has no documentation of vaccination on or after his or her first birthday, laboratory verification of the diseases, or physician-diagnosed infection. People who were immunized between 1963 and 1967 with the killed measles alone or the killed measles vaccine followed by the live type should be revaccinated. Further if the type of vaccine is unknown, the individual should be revaccinated. Inclusion of live rubella virus can be risky for the fetus of women becoming pregnant within 3 months of immunization.

Tuberculosis

Control of tuberculosis is generally aimed at means other than immunization in the United States. These measures include early detection, treatment with various anti-tuberculosis drugs, or prevention therapy using the agent isoniazid. However, main strains are resistant to various drugs, and there are areas where the likelihood of infection is high. In those instances, vaccination with BCG, bacille Calmette-Guerin, should be considered for dental personnel. BCG contains a weakened strain of the tubercle bacillus. The suggested administration is a single dose of 0.3 mL given percutaneously under the skin. Pregnant women, or individuals who are immunocompromised, such as those with HIV or various cancers, should not be given the vaccine.

Preventing Adverse Reactions

Latex allergies

Use of non-latex gloves is the best way to prevent dental worker exposure, but powder-free or reduced-protein latex gloves do cut down on potential exposure. It is recommended that the dental office follow the recommendations of the National Institute for Occupational Safety and Health, discussed in detail elsewhere. It is very important to determine whether patients might be allergic to latex or rubber products by including in their medical history a number of relevant questions. The medical history of the patient should include information about allergies to rubber-containing products ranging from balloons to condoms, allergies to certain foods such as bananas and kiwis, possible exposure through surgical procedures at any time in their life, allergic testing results if performed, presence of asthma or hay fever, and current use of rubber gloves or other latex-containing products. Special precautions should be taken for patients with possible latex allergies. They should be treated at the beginning of the day in a room in which latex is excluded before and during treatment. This exclusion includes anything in contact with the patient, anything a dental worker is wearing, and possible airborne latex proteins from glove powder.

<u>Possible harmful reactions to gloves</u>

Latex is derived from the rubber tree *Hevea brasiliensis*. The latex goes through quite a bit of processing and other materials are added to make gloves. Up to 6% of the populace and 12% of regularly exposed healthcare workers may be sensitive to latex. Most reactions to latex gloves are actually to other chemicals in the gloves or put on the hands in the form of irritant contact dermatitis. There are two forms of true allergic reactions to latex possible as well, allergic contact dermatitis and latex allergy. Allergic contact dermatitis is a delayed type IV hypersensitivity reaction to latex in gloves or often the chemicals used during processing of them. It is characterized by itching, erythema, and vesicles a day or two after exposure and later dry skin, cracks, and sores. The other type, latex allergy, is type I hypersensitivity elicited by substances released upon exposure to latex proteins by mast cells to which IgE class anti-latex antibodies are bound. Signs of latex allergic appear rapidly about 20 minutes after exposure and can include hives, erythema, sneezing, and asthma. Allergic individuals with subsequent exposures can go into anaphylactic shock and possibly die. Latex allergy can be elicited by airborne latex proteins from glove powder.

<u>NIOSH recommendations for prevention of latex allergies</u>

The National Institute for Occupational Safety and Health (NIOSH) has issued recommendations for workers and employers for prevention of latex allergies in the workplace. The NIOSH recommends that workers use nonlatex gloves when appropriate or at least use latex gloves that are powder-free with reduced protein or refrain from use of oil- or petroleum-based lotions, which degrade the gloves. If latex gloves are used, the worker should wash and dry hands after removal. An office utilizing latex gloves requires frequent cleaning including changing of ventilation filters and vacuum bags. The personnel should be informed about ways to prevent latex allergies and the potential signs. Individuals should refrain from use of latex-containing gloves and other articles if they have symptoms of latex allergy. If they have symptoms of latex allergy, they should confer with a physician. Latex-allergic personnel should wear a medical alert bracelet stating that fact. The employer's responsibilities include provision of nonlatex and/or reduced-protein, powder-free gloves, institution of housekeeping procedures that get rid of latex dust, offering education regarding latex allergy, regular evaluation of personnel for latex allergy symptoms, and ongoing quality control.

Standard/Universal Precautions and the Prevention of Disease Transmission

Hand hygiene

At the onset of the working day, the worker should remove jewelry and cleanse the hands, nails and forearms with a liquid antimicrobial agent and soft brush for 15 seconds. The worker should then rinse by rubbing with cool or tepid water for 10 seconds, dry all areas with clean paper towels, and shut off the faucet with a paper towel. The worker should also practice routine hand hygiene throughout the day. This can be lathering with a liquid non-antimicrobial or antimicrobial soap for 15 seconds followed by 10 second rinsing, drying and turning off the faucet as described previously. Use of non-antimicrobial soaps gets rid of soil and transient microbial flora, but use of antimicrobial soaps also reduces resident skin flora. Alternatively, if there is no soiling visible, alcohol-based hand rubbing agents can be used by putting them in the palm of the hand and rubbing. Hand hygiene should be performed at the beginning and end of the day, anytime hands are soiled, anytime bare hands are in contact with contaminated surfaces or objects, before and after use of gloves, after using the restroom, and prior to activities such as eating, applying makeup, or handling contacts.

The certified dental assistant should carry out hand hygiene thoroughly with soap and water for one minute on arrival at work, and thereafter with soap and water (if hands are visibly soiled) or alcohol rub whenever the hands are contaminated, before applying gloves, before and after assisting patients, and after removing gloves. Antimicrobial soaps are only recommended if the hands have had contact with blood or body fluids. Note that any lotions applied to the hands should be compatible with latex. Jewelry and artificial nails should be avoided as they may harbor bacteria. Hand hygiene procedure:

- Wet hands thoroughly with warm water, apply soap, and rub hands together to massage the soap into the tissue, including between the fingers and about the nails.
- Rinse hands completely to remove all soap.
- Dry hands completely with clean towel or air dry.
- Use a clean towel or foot control to turn off the water.

If using alcohol rub, it should be thoroughly rubbed into all surfaces for at least 15 seconds. Drying time should take at least 15 seconds or insufficient rub was applied.

<u>Antimicrobial spectrum of commonly used hand hygiene agents</u>

Hand hygiene agents are designed to remove transient skin flora, microorganisms to which an individual is exposed when touching contaminated areas. Transient skin flora differs from normal resident skin flora in that transient flora is less deeply embedded and potentially more dangerous. Alcohol-based hand rubs containing 60 to 90% alcohol are the fastest acting and are quite effective against all potential pathogens, including gram-positive and negative bacteria, mycobacterium, fungi and viruses. Intermediate in terms of speed of action are chlorhexidine (2 or 4%), iodophors, phenolics and triclosan. All of these are fairly effective against bacteria. Of these, chlorhexidine is the reagent with the broadest spectrum of effectiveness against other types of microorganisms, it continues to be effective longer, and it rarely produces allergic reactions. Quaternary ammonium compounds act slowly, are only used in conjunction with alcohols, and they are only minimally effective against bacteria and viruses. Mycobacteria and fungi are resistant to triclosan and quaternary ammonium compounds.

Alcohol-based hand rubs

Alcohol-based hand rubs are very effective for hand hygiene and asepsis. Unfortunately they are also flammable because most contain at least 60% isopropyl or ethyl alcohol. It is the opinion of the American Society of Healthcare Engineering that alcohol-based hand rub dispensers can be located in hallways, suites, or near patient room entries with the following restrictions. The largest single containers of gel/liquid alcohol-based rubs that can be used are 1.2 liters in egress corridors and 2 liters in suites such as dental operatories. The dispensers cannot be mounted anywhere near electric receptacles or other possible ignition sources. If the container extends more than 3.5 inches into a corridor, it should be documented in the fire plan and training program. Alcohol-based hand rub containers being stored must be in an official flammable liquid storage cabinet. Total amounts of alcohol-based hand rubs present in the facility should not surpass amounts indicated by building and fire codes.

Hand hygiene prior to surgical procedures

Prior to surgical procedures, Jewelry is removed and multiple scrub and rinse cycles (from 2 to 6 minutes) using either an antimicrobial surgical scrub product or a non-antimicrobial agent are done. This is followed by rinsing and keeping the hands above the elbow level. The person lets water drip off from the elbows and then dries the hands with sterile towels. If an antimicrobial surgical scrub product, which eliminates soil and transient flora and kills some resident microbes as well, was used, the person then puts on sterile gloves with the aid of an assistant. If a non-antimicrobial agent was used, then an alcohol-based hand rub should be rubbed into the hand before sterile gloves are donned as previously described. In both cases, the gloves must be vigorously inspected for defects and no contaminated surfaces or other items should be touched.

Personal Protective Equipment (PPE)

Donning and removing personal protective equipment

There is a suggested sequence for use of personal protective equipment. Protective clothing should be donned before performing activities such as positioning the patient's bib and unpacking instruments and supplies. Then the worker puts on the mask and eyewear. Prior to treatment procedures, the worker should wash his or her hands as described elsewhere and don gloves. No contaminated surfaces should be handled once gloves are donned prior to patient contact. When procedures are completed, the suggested sequence of PPE removal is disposable gown if used, then gloves, followed by protective eyewear, and the mask. This sequence of removal is performed by pulling the gown off over gloves turning it inside out, taking off the first glove with the other hand by pinching at the wrist and pulling in the direction of the fingers, and then placing the ungloved thumb inside the wrist area of the other glove and pulling in off toward the fingers. Eyewear and the mask are subsequently removed by grasping the ear rests and elastic bands or ties respectively.

Gloves used in dentistry

The two main types of gloves used in dentistry are those for patient care activities and those designed as utility gloves. There are also specialized types such as heat-resistant gloves (for use with sterilizers, etc.) and cotton dermal gloves. No matter what type of patient care gloves are employed, they should be disposable and used for a single patient or until compromised (cuts, tears). Patient care gloves are either sterile for surgical procedures or non-sterile for all other routines. They can also be categorized according to material. Gloves may be made of latex or some other material. Many people are allergic to latex. Sterile patient care surgical gloves come in latex, reduced-protein latex, neoprene, styrene, and synthetic copolymers. Examination gloves are generally latex, synthetic copolymer, nitrile, styrene-butadiene, or polyurethane. Latex gloves also come in powderless, flavored, and low-protein versions. Utility gloves should be worn during cleaning activities, preparation and use of chemicals, and instrument processing. Utility gloves are heavier, made of materials like heavy latex or nitrile and in some instances thin copolymer or plastic. Each worker should have his or her own assigned pair, which should be washed with an antimicrobial agent, rinsed, and dried.

Role of glove use in infection control

Gloves are one aspect of personal protective equipment (PPE). According the OSHA Bloodborne Pathogens Standard gloves must be provided in facilities such as dental offices where workers may be exposed to bloodborne pathogens. Gloves used in the dental office protect members of the dental team from infections transmitted by patients, patients from infections spread by the dental team, and patients from infections from other patients. Dentists and other members of the dental team who wear gloves have a barrier to transmission from the patient though cuts in their skin. Gloves also protect dental personnel against irritants like chemicals and dental materials. Certain gloves guard against burns during processing operations. Donning of gloves during patient operations by the dentist and other personnel protects the patient from microorganisms on the worker's hands. Dental workers can be in contact with infectious agents on just about every contaminated surface in the area, and they may harbor bloodborne pathogens that can escape through cuts on the skin. If they are in contact with patient's blood it can be preserved on the hands for days, particularly under fingernails, and spread to other patients if ungloved.

Protective eyewear

Protective eyewear is a form of personal protective equipment (PPE). It comes in a variety of forms, including goggles (the best coverage), prescription eyeglasses that have side shields, and protective eyeglasses with shields. There are also masks with attached eye protection and face shields. Protective eyewear serves two purposes. It protects the mucous membranes in the eye from exposure to potentially infectious sprays, splatters, or aerosols. It also offers protection against impact damage to the eyes which can occur during activities such as polishing or grinding, chemical splashes, and ultraviolet irradiation. Therefore, protective eyewear use is suggested for a variety of activities in the dental office, including grinding and polishing materials, cleaning instruments or surfaces, developing radiographs and working in the dental lab.

Masks

Masks are personal protective equipment (PPE). They are classified according to the level of bacterial or particle filter efficiency as N-series (95%), R-series (99%) or P-series (99.97%). In dentistry, the primary purpose of face masks is to protect the dental worker's nasal and oral mucous membranes against sprays, splatters, or aerosolized particles from the patient that could contain infectious agents. The masks also reduce worker to patient transmission. Masks should be worn and then discarded after single patient use during certain procedures. These procedures include anything involving handpieces, ultrasonic scalers, air/water syringes, and oral irrigators. Face mask use is also suggested during polishing or grinding of potentially contaminated items (for example in the dental lab) and during instrument processing. Since masks are dome shaped or flat covering the bridge of the nose, they can allow some transmission of fluids or aerosols if they are not tight. Thus respirators instead of masks are indicated in some instances such as when treating patients with potential airborne infections such as SARS (severe acute respiratory syndrome).

Protective clothing

Protective clothing should be donned over street clothes by dental workers anytime there is potential for splashing or spraying of blood, saliva, or other potentially infectious materials. Examples of acceptable protective clothing include lab coats, gowns, uniforms, aprons and jackets. Clothing that resists fluids is preferable. Disposable protective gowns are useful; they should be discarded in biohazardous waste daily or when soiled. Reusable protective garments should also be taken off when soiled and anytime the worker leaves the office. OSHA requires that reusable protective clothing be left at the office and be laundered there or through a commercial laundering service. Work shoes to be worn only at the workplace are another form of protective clothing; these are not mandated by law.

Instrument processing area

The instrument processing area should be distinct from other spaces, yet centrally located. Ideally it should be in a separate room or rooms with no outside doors or windows to let in dust and good ventilation. There should be three separate areas for decontamination, packaging, and sterilizing and storage. There should be a logical work flow within each zone and between zones. Each area should be clearly marked. The decontamination area should be equipped with personal protective equipment, a sharps container, tongs, a sink and handwashing dispenser, an ultrasonic cleaner and detergent, waste containers for biohazardous materials and nonregulated waste, facilities to prepare handpieces (cleaners, lubricants, air and vacuum lines for flushing), and a drainer. The packaging area should be equipped with rust inhibitors, replacement parts, biologic and chemical indicators, packaging materials, a heat sealer, and autoclave tape. The sterilizing should contain the sterilizer(s), appropriate solutions (water, glutaraldehyde, etc.), a glutaraldehyde monitor if used, lubricant for the handpiece, air and vacuum lines for flushing excess lubricant, an incubator for culturing spore strips/vials, and an enclosed storage space.

Protecting the Patient and the Operator

Universal and standard precautions

Universal precautions are infection control measures needed to prevent exposure to blood and other bodily fluids of patients, who are treated as if they are infectious. Standard precautions are more inclusive infection control measures that extend to blood, all bodily fluids such as secretions and excretions (excluding sweat), skin that is not intact, and mucous membranes. All of these are considered as potentially infectious under standard precautions because even if patients exhibit no symptoms they can be asymptomatic carriers of disease agents. Wording in the OSHA Bloodborne Pathogens Standard still refers to universal precautions, but the more inclusive standard precautions should be followed in the dental office.

Protective barriers

All appropriate personal protective equipment (PPE) should be available, utilized by the employee whenever there is potential exposure to patient blood or saliva or contaminated surfaces, and removed once the employee leaves the area. PPE includes gloves, masks, protective eyewear, and protective clothing. All of these pieces of equipment should be cleaned regularly or, if appropriate, discarded. Many types of gloves and other items should be available to deal with possible adverse reactions, especially latex allergy, which patients should be questioned about. Employees whose duties necessitate using gloves should have short fingernails, refrain from using petrolatum or oil-based lotions, and use nonlatex or low latex versions if reactions are a concern. Nonsterile gloves are appropriate except during surgical procedures when sterile surgeon's gloves should be worn. If reusable protective clothing is worn, it should be put in a designated container (biohazard symbol, color coded) when contaminated and either laundered at the office or sent to a laundry service, never taken home.

Dental dams and eye shields

A dental dam is a rubber or silicone barrier that is placed in the mouth to separate the site of dental treatment from the rest of the mouth. The dam helps to keep saliva away from the operative site so that it remains clean and dry, allows improved visibility, protects soft tissue in the mouth, and decreases risk of the patient inadvertently swallowing dental debris. For procedures, such as root canals, the use of a dental dam is an infection control procedure. However, the dental dam prevents the patient from communicating while it's in place. Patients are unable to breathe through the mouth with the dam in place, so they must be able to breathe through the nose. Some patients may not be able to tolerate use of the dam because it makes them feel claustrophobic. Eye shields should be used by both the patient and the operator (who should also wear a facemask) during any drilling procedure in which there may be spray or other aerosolized debris to protect the eyes from contamination and injury.

Saliva ejectors

Saliva ejectors are used to suction saliva and fluids out of the oral cavity during procedures. Studies indicate that there is a great likelihood of a reverse flow in the vacuum line back into the patient's mouth if a seal is created around the saliva ejector. This reverse flow could transmit infectious agents. Therefore, measures to prevent the retraction are suggested. The patient should be instructed to refrain from closing the lips tightly around the ejector. Another way to ensure against creating a seal and inducing retraction is to use disposable saliva ejector tips that have a tiny hole on the side, which reduces pressure and stops reverse flow.

Pre-procedure mouth rinse

Pre-procedure mouth rinsing by the patient with an antimicrobial mouth rinse greatly reduces the number of microorganisms in the oral cavity. Thus, fewer oral microbes can be transmitted during procedures as aerosols, splatter, or directly through contact to the professional. This should also reduce surface contamination in the area. It is particularly suggested that a patient do a mouth rinse before procedures involving a prophylaxis cup or ultrasonic scaler as these practices preclude use of other aseptic measures such as a rubber dam and high-volume evacuation. In addition, it is beneficial for dental team members to use a long-lasting antimicrobial mouth rinse, generally containing chlorhexidine gluconate, essential oils, and ionosphere.

Prevent Cross-Contamination During Procedures

Aseptic techniques

Aseptic techniques are any procedures that reduce or eliminate the dissemination of pathogens. One of the most basic aseptic techniques is ensuring that one touches as few surfaces as possible with the fingers (gloved or ungloved) that might be coated with blood or saliva. This can be accomplished by making sure that surfaces are covered or cleaned and disinfected. Gloves are used but changed every time they are contaminated or the professional leaves the chair side. The professional should avoid touching his or her person with contaminated, gloved hands. Another important aseptic technique is the reduction of dental aerosols and spatter produced by use of handpieces, ultrasonic scalers and the air/water syringe. This can be accomplished through methods such as the use of high-volume evacuation (HVE) and a rubber dam. The HVE system should also be cleaned by flushing with detergent or detergent-disinfectant combination at the conclusion of each day and emptying the trap periodically. The rubber dam isolates the area being worked on and minimizes saliva. Other techniques include pre-procedure mouth rinsing, use of disposables whenever possible, and effective housekeeping.

General methods and aseptic techniques as part of infection control program

Standard precautions should always be followed. Other general methods include proper hand hygiene, avoidance of activities like eating and applying cosmetics in the area, having the patient rinse his or her mouth before a procedure, measures to diminish splattering of blood or saliva, never using disposables for more than one patient, and checking of sterilized instrument packages prior to use. Dental water is an important consideration. It should contain less than 500 CFU/mL of heterotrophic bacteria. It should not be used to irrigate surgical sites. Its ant retraction valves should always be in order, and all devices connected to it should be flushed for 20 to 30 seconds between patients.

Housekeeping and cleaning techniques to minimize dust and microorganisms

In addition to surface disinfection and sterilization procedures discussed elsewhere, there are general housekeeping considerations. Dusting and sweeping in any patient care locales should be done with wet cloths or mops to reduce dispersal of microorganism-containing dust. These cloths and mops should be disposable or they should be permitted to dry between uses. The mop water should contain a low-level disinfectant, for example, a quaternary ammonium compound, and it should be changed at least every day. During periods when the office is closed, dust covers might be utilized for surfaces in the operatory and sterilizing rooms. Filters need to be replaced often. Patient care areas should have smooth surface floors (not carpeting) and no cloth upholstery. Other office areas should be kept clean and dust-free.

Infection control procedures upon completion of dental treatment

At the completion of a dental treatment, the dental assistant should remove handpieces and tips for the HVE and air/water syringe while still gloved. He or she should then don overgloves to document information on the patient's chart or in the computer, gather radiographs, and remove the patient's napkin. After dismissing the patient, the assistant while gloved should put the handpiece, HVE, and air/water syringe back on the unit and flush them. Afterwards the handpiece and syringe are placed back on the treatment tray. Sharps are carefully placed into the sharps container, and the chair cover is removed by inversion to create a bag. This bag conformation will contain potential infectious material within. Subsequently barriers and disposables are removed and placed within the bag. The assistant should then carry the treatment tray to the sterilizing area before removing gloves and putting them in the bag, which is properly disposed of. At the end, the assistant should wash his or her hands.

Disinfection and cleaning of final treatment room

After a patient has been treated and dismissed and other post-treatment procedures are performed, the dental assistant should wash his or her hands and don utility gloves. Surfaces are then disinfected with an intermediate level disinfectant following an established routine. Iodophors, sodium hypochlorite (bleach), and phenolics qualify as intermediate level disinfectants. All necessary solutions, towels, and 4 x 4 gauze squares are carried into the area. All surfaces are sprayed with the disinfectant, wiped to get rid of debris, sprayed again and left for about 10 minutes, and then wiped off again. Alternatively, gauze squares can be sprayed with disinfectant and used to wipe down the surfaces. It is important to remember to disinfect surfaces like the chair adjustments, amalgam cradle, view box, and curing light all of which are potentially contaminated.

Clinical contact surfaces and housekeeping surfaces

Clinical contact surfaces are any surfaces predisposed to contamination during patient care activities. They might be touched with gloved hands during patient care or in some other way become contaminated with potentially infectious materials. Examples of clinical contact surfaces are as follows: various controls and switches; countertops; hoses connected to the handpiece, evacuator or air/water syringe; various parts of the x-ray unit; the chair back or headrest; the handle and tip of the light curing instrument, mirror and faucet handles; and shade guides. Some clinical contact surfaces such as controls, handles and the light curing tip should be protected with surface covers while others must be precleaned and disinfected. Housekeeping surfaces are those surfaces that do not generally come in contact with contaminated hands or devices such as floors, walls and basin. These surfaces can be treated at the conclusion of the day while clinical contact surfaces need to be addressed more immediately.

Protecting against surface contamination

Surfaces that are non-electrical, smooth, and easily reached are appropriately treated with precleaning and disinfection as opposed to using surface covers. Precleaning reduces the bioburden. Soap and water or preferably a surface cleaner/disinfectant is used for the precleaning step. There are two accepted methods for precleaning and disinfection. Utility gloves and personal protective equipment should be worn during either process. The first method is the spray-wipe-spray technique in which the surface is initially sprayed with cleaning/disinfecting agent, thoroughly wiped with paper towels, resprayed with disinfectant agent, and left moist for about 10 minutes. This method can be done using paper towels or gauze pads saturated with the disinfecting agent instead of spraying. The other method is the wipe-discard-wipe technique in which a disinfectant towelette from a dispenser is used to wipe the surface, discarded, another towelette is used to wipe the surface again and discarded, and the surface is allowed to dry. In either case, if the surface is wet when needed for patient care, it can be wiped dry. Disinfectant should be rinsed or wiped off surfaces that will come in contact with the patient's mouth or skin.

Intermediate-level disinfectants

Intermediate-level disinfectants are used for disinfection of clinical contact surfaces and noncritical surfaces laden with visible blood. The most commonly used intermediate-level agents are chlorine compounds, iodophors, alcohols, synthetic phenolics, and quaternary ammonium compounds. Theoretically these should only be used in forms that are EPA-registered and claim to have tuberculocidal activity. The main chloride compound used is sodium hypochlorite as part of an EPA-registered product, or commercial bleach diluted freshly 1:10 to 1:100. Iodophors are iodine-containing compounds. They may be corrosive and/or staining and generally require dilution before use. Ethyl or isopropyl alcohols are usually used in combination these days with phenolics. Phenol or carbolic acid is quite toxic, but synthetic phenolics incorporating phenol are not; they usually come in combination with another phenolic or an alcohol. Quaternary ammonium compounds are cationic detergents and are only tuberculocidal, intermediate-level agents when in combination with alcohol, which augments antimicrobial activity.

Decontamination of all equipment used in patient care area

First of all, disposables should be used and discarded afterwards whenever possible, regardless of whether or not the equipment penetrates soft tissue or tooth structure. Non-disposable instruments that penetrate soft tissue or tooth structure should be cleaned, packaged, and heat sterilized after use. Non-disposable instruments that are used in the mouth but do not pierce soft teeth tissue or tooth structure should be treated in various ways depending on whether they can be covered and whether they are heat stable. If they can be covered, that is the method of choice. Items such as these include the handle of a mouth mirror or a light-curing tip. If they cannot be covered, the approach depends on whether or not they are heat stable. Items that can withstand high temperatures should be packaged and heat sterilized while those that are heat-sensitive should be sterilized in a liquid sterilant, rinsed, and packaged. Equipment in the area that is susceptible to contamination via splatter or touch but not directly used in the patient's mouth should be heat sterilized if possible. If the equipment cannot be sterilized, it should be covered to thwart contamination or cleaned and disinfected. If there is little chance of contamination of room items, for example the walls, they can simply be cleaned.

Infection control considerations for digital radiography and other high-tech equipment

Reusable intraoral sensors are utilized with digital radiography. Infection control depends on the type of sensor used. A CCD or charge-coupled device sensor and its attached cable should be covered with a plastic barrier to prevent contamination. CCD sensors are heat-sensitive and should never be heat sterilized, but they can be disinfected by the spray-wipe-spray method is contamination occurs. Complementary metal-oxide semiconductor with active pixel sensors should be treated similarly. Photostimulable phosphor plate sensors must be covered thoroughly with plastic barriers as they cannot withstand heat sterilization or disinfection. Computers should either be used with clean hands or, if contaminated, swabbed with disinfectant wipes. Cameras cannot be decontaminated and therefore should be covered with plastic or used only with clean hands. Computer-aided design or manufacturing devices (CAD/CAMS) have a small camera and wire that is placed in a patient's mouth; here manufacturer's directions for decontamination should be followed.

Surface covers

If surface covers are impermeable to fluids and thick enough to resist tearing, they are appropriate for protection against surface contamination by blood, saliva, or other possibly contaminated fluids. Various types of plastic covers generally meet the requirements. Specially fitted covers, plastic sheets and plastic bags are used in various combinations. Surface covers should be put on before surfaces are exposed to contamination. Otherwise the surface must first be precleaned and disinfected while gloved, the gloves discarded, and hands washed before placing the covers. The surface covers should be removed with gloved hands at the end of patient care or other activities. Care should be taken not to touch the surface under the cover during removal, and if the surface is touched, precleaning and disinfection must be done as above. Used covers can be thrown into the standard trash unless local legislation deems them regulated waste. Afterwards contaminated gloves should be discarded, hands washed, and new surface covers applied before the next patient. Surface covers are not appropriate for some surfaces such as the bracket table, countertops, and mirror hands all of which are usually precleaned and disinfected.

Laboratory and radiographic asepsis

The primary consideration in terms of laboratory asepsis is that any item that has been contaminated with oral fluids should ideally be sterilized; if that is impossible, the item should at least be rinsed and disinfected prior to being sent to the dental laboratory. In turn, items sent from the dental laboratory to the office should be disinfected, rinsed, confirmed as such, and established as being uncontaminated before they are inserted into a patient's mouth. The major tactic in terms of radiographic asepsis is the covering of x-ray films and digital x-ray sensors with plastic surface covers before they are inserted into the patient's mouth. If films or sensors are not covered with plastic barriers, then they must be rinsed and disinfected or handled aseptically after removal. Also, if daylight loaders are used, then caution must be exercised to avoid contact between contaminated gloves or films and the loader's sleeves.

Infection control procedures prior to and during radiographic exposure

The dental assistant should wash his or her hands and place all barriers, which are generally various plastic covers or bags, on all equipment and possibly other surfaces. Alternatively, surfaces could be disinfected if shorting of equipment is not an issue. Barriers such as sandwich bags should be placed on either side of the lead-lined x-ray room door and switches. Often chairs are covered as well. Dental films to be exposed should be placed within FDA-cleared plastic, protective barrier pouches. If digital radiographic sensors are utilized for digital radiography instead of films, they should be protected with disposable plastic covers (preferably FDA-cleared). Generally, complete personal protective equipment is donned when the patient is seated. Disposable or heat-tolerant film holders that can be sterilized between patients should be used. After each x-ray is exposed, it is placed in a disposable cup before transportation for processing. Barriers and gloves are removed after patient procedures are completed; they are generally not considered regulated medical waste but local regulations for disposal should be considered. Exposed surfaces should be disinfected.

Infection control procedures related to processing of radiographs

Exposed x-ray films should be conveyed to the darkroom in disposable cups or within a paper towel. There the dental assistant (wearing disposable gloves) should drop each film out of its packet onto an uncontaminated, disposable paper towel or into a cup. After all are removed, he or she then discards the packets and gloves, washes hands, and starts the processing procedure. For processing, gloves should be worn anytime films are contaminated. So for manual processing, gloves should be donned if the films were not protected during exposure with removable protective film pouches, but they are also generally necessary because films are dunked into solutions. If automatic processing with a daylight loader is done, films must first be placed inside the loader and unwrapped and dropped into another cup or paper towel inside the loader while gloved (powder-free gloves recommended). The waste is collected in another cup and the dental assistant then inserts each opened film into the automatic processor with bare hands. Alternatively, he or she might initially use overgloves, which are removed for insertion.

Laboratory asepsis during operation of dental lathe

A dental lathe is used in the dental laboratory to grind, polish, and blast prostheses and impressions for proper presentation. Its use creates many opportunities for injuries as well as the spread of microorganisms. Protective eyewear, preferably with a front Plexiglas shield, should always be worn when using a dental lathe. The room should be adequately ventilated, and mask use is suggested as well. The spread of infectious agents can be facilitated by techniques such as the following: use of the lathe through hand holes, creating a barrier; sterilization or disinfection of all accessories; disinfection of the unit twice daily; and utilization of new pumice and pan liners for each item. Polishing agents should always be discarded if unused, not returned to their source. Disposable polishing attachments should be used if possible; if not, they should be sterilized or disinfected between uses as directed.

Handpiece asepsis

The inside and outside of handpieces and their attachments must be cleaned and sterilized between patients as they may contain patient materials. While still attached to the hose after patient treatment, the handpiece should be wiped free of visible debris. High-speed handpieces should also be flushed 20 to 30 seconds into the vacuum line or some receptacle like the sink or a container. The handpiece is then removed from the hose and externally cleaned, rinsed and dried. Then the internal parts should be cleaned and lubricated per manufacturer's instructions. The handpiece is reconnected to the air/water system for flushing the excess out as before. Surplus lubricant on the outside is wiped off. At that point, the handpiece should be packaged and sterilized as directed by the manufacturer. Note that some handpieces cannot withstand extremely high temperatures such as those used in dry heat sterilizers. The handpiece is then dried, cooled, and retained in the packaging until ready for use. Some handpieces need post-sterilization lubrication; if so, using aseptic technique the bag is opened, lubricant is squirted into it, the hose is attached, and excess lubricant is extruded.

Disinfection

Disinfection is the use of chemical agents called disinfectants that can destroy most microorganisms but not the more resistant bacteria or fungal spores. Disinfectants are generally used at room temperature to reduce microbial load on surfaces. Chemicals that are used for disinfection include agents such as iodophors, phenolics, sodium hypochlorite, alcohol, and quaternary ammonium compounds. Some high-level disinfectants such as glutaraldehyde can also be used for liquid chemical sterilization if used for prolonged periods. Unlike some methods of sterilization, there is no way of monitoring the effectiveness of surface disinfection.

Chemicals that can kill microorganisms

There are four types of chemicals that can destroy microorganisms. Two of these types are only effective in or on the body. These are antibiotics, which are effective only systemically or topically, and antiseptics, which are chemicals that effective in killing microorganisms on the skin or other body surfaces but should not be used systemically. The other two types are utilized only on inanimate surfaces, sterilants or disinfectants. A sterilant is a chemical that can kill all microorganisms on inanimate objects including most bacterial spores. Disinfectants are chemicals that can destroy various types of microorganisms on environmental surfaces or inanimate objects but usually not high numbers of bacterial spores.

Categories of disinfecting or sterilizing chemicals

The Centers for Disease Control classifies disinfectants by their spectrum of activity against microbial agents. The organization groups sterilants and high-level disinfectants together. Both destroy all microorganisms on submerged, inanimate, heat-sensitive items but only sterilants also destroy most bacterial spores. The chemicals falling into both these categories are glutaraldehyde, glutaraldehyde-hydephenate, hydrogen peroxide with or without peracetic acid, and peracetic acid. Another chemical, orthophthalaldehyde, is strictly a high-level disinfectant. Intermediate-level disinfectants can kill vegetative bacteria and most fungi and viruses and inactivate *Mycobacterium tuberculosis* var *bovis* on surfaces. EPA-registered hospital disinfectants claiming tuberculocidal activity fall into this category. They contain phenolics, iodophors, and quaternary ammonium compounds plus alcohol, bromides, or chlorides. Low-level disinfectants destroy vegetative bacteria and some fungi and viruses but are not tuberculocidal. Low-level hospital disinfectants are generally quaternary ammonium compounds; they should be used only for housekeeping surfaces unless they claim reactivity against HIV and HBV.

Terms commonly found on labeling for antimicrobial products

Terms with the suffix "-cidal" indicate that the agent has at least some ability to kill a particular type of microorganism. Thus the terms "bactericidal", "virucidal", or "fungicidal" mean the agent can destroy at least some bacteria, viruses, or fungi respectively. More specific activity is indicated by the terms "tuberculocidal" or "sporicidal," which refer to the ability to kill *Mycobacterium tuberculosis* var *bovis* or bacterial spores respectively. An agent that is sporicidal is essentially a sterilant. Labels often specify the genus and species of microorganisms they can kill as well in addition to other information about the product. If a label brands the product as a hospital disinfectant, it indicates that it has been demonstrated to destroy the bacterial species *Staphylococcus aureus, Salmonella choleraesuis,* and *Pseudomonas aeruginosa.*

Warning labels used on potentially infectious containers

Regulated waste, refrigerators, freezers, sharps, or any other containers used for transport must be labeled with the word "Biohazard" on a fluorescent orange or orange-red label. There is usually also a biohazard symbol on the label made up of interconnected circular patterns. Individual unlabeled containers of potentially infectious materials can be placed within labeled ones. If employees are clearly informed, alternatives can include red bags or containers. Contaminated equipment being transported must be labeled as well, including the area of contamination. Contaminated laundry that is sent offsite should generally be bagged and labeled similarly unless the laundry facility is known to use universal precautions (they should still be clearly identified). Contaminated sharps need to be discarded into leak proof, puncture-resistant, closable, and red and/or "Biohazard" labeled containers. Other regulated waste that might be infectious should be put in leakproof, closable, color-coded or labeled containers such as biohazard bags.

Disposal procedures for blood in liquid or semiliquid form

Blood in free-flowing liquid or semiliquid form is regarded as an infectious and regulated medical waste. The Centers for Disease Control (CDC) recommends that blood, suctioned fluids, and other liquid waste be decanted carefully down a drain connected to a sanitary sewer system. This method of disposal should only be employed if it is in compliance with local and state regulations as well. There may be restrictions aimed at minimizing the volume of blood in the sewage system. If blood is disposed of in the water system, daily rinsing of sink traps and evacuation lines with a nonbleach disinfectant and water is recommended.

Types of waste generated in dental offices

Medical waste is any solid waste produced during diagnosis, treatment, or immunization in some type of healthcare facility. Most medical waste is not infectious and is not regulated. Items that have touched blood or other bodily fluids are considered contaminated waste, and wastes that can place a human being or the environment at risk are deemed hazardous. Infectious waste is the portion of medical waste that is capable of inducing an infectious disease. Infectious waste is a regulated medical waste governed by the OSHA Bloodborne Pathogens Standard. There are 5 types of OSHA regulated medical waste, all of which can be found in dentistry. These 5 categories are blood or other potentially infectious material (OPIM) such as saliva in liquid or semiliquid form, contaminated items that could discharge the same if compressed, articles caked with dried blood or OPIM that could liberate infectious materials, contaminated sharps, and pathologic or microbiologic wastes that contain OPIM or blood. Another waste classification is toxic waste, which is refuse that can be poisonous.

Sharps safety and disposal

Sharps (for example, needles, scalpel blades, and broken glass) are regarded as infectious and regulated as medical waste. OSHA mandates that disposable sharps be put in sharps containers directly after use. Sharps containers must be clearly-marked (biohazard symbol, color-coded usually red), leakproof, closable, and puncture-resistant. There are many ways to make sharps use safer. In particular, when using injection needles, one should either use some sort of protective cap-holding contrivance or the cap sheath should be replaced using the one-handed scoop method. Other safety measures include organizing sharp instruments and handpieces with tips or burs pointing away from the operator, filling sharps containers to a maximum of three-quarters full, and use of tongs or pliers to pick up sharps or disengage burs. When sharps containers are full, they can be relayed to waste handlers or, if allowed by state law, decontaminated onsite in a steam sterilizer. In the latter case, "sterilizable" sharps containers should be at most ¾ full. They are placed upright with vents open into the sterilizer and autoclaved for 40 to 60 minutes, cooled, closed, labeled, and disposed of in a manner allowed locally.

Disposal procedures for pathogenic waste

In the dental office, pathogenic waste consists of biopsy specimens, excised tissues, and most often, extracted teeth that are not returned to the patient. All of these are considered OSHA regulated wastes that are potentially infectious. They should be placed in leakproof, color-coded containers, either biohazard bags or in the case of teeth possibly sharps containers. After collection, pathogenic waste should be decontaminated or neutralized in a steam autoclave or chemical vapor sterilizer before boxing and discarding the treated waste according to local regulations. Extracted teeth that contain amalgam restorations should be disinfected with full-strength glutaraldehyde or another sterilizing chemical instead of any type of heat sterilization. CDC recommendations also permit return of extracted teeth to the patient.

Management of regulated waste

Regulated waste includes sharps, nonsharps waste, liquids to be disposed of, and human tissues (such as teeth). Each type of waste should be handled, processed, and stored in a proper manner, and containers should be clearly labeled with a biohazard symbol, color coding, and if necessary, name and address. Sharps are a major concern. They should be handled carefully. Sharps containers should be readily available and never overfilled. Specimens containing human tissue or any bodily fluid including blood should be put in appropriate containers and clearly labeled with a biohazard symbol and color coding. **Regulations regarding processing of regulated waste should be followed prior to their being discarded or transported to a disposal facility.** Records should be kept documenting the treatment, transport, and disposal of regulated waste.

Instrument/Device Processing

Processing of Reusable Dental Instruments

Instrument processing

Reusable sharps should be carefully placed after use in labeled containers (biohazard symbol, color coded) that can be secured for transport. There should be a main instrument processing area with separate sections for cleaning and decontamination, packaging, and sterilization, and storage. Handpieces and their attachments and reusable instruments must be sterilized between patients. Contaminated instruments should be mechanically cleaned, rinsed, dried, packaged for sterilization, and sterilized using the appropriate technique. Most instruments should be sterilized in a steam sterilizer or autoclave, but if they are more heat-sensitive, a low-temperature process such as soaking in glutaraldehyde can be used. Sterilizers should undergo spore testing weekly (and records kept) as well as monitored for correct timing and temperature. Packages should have an attached temperature strip that indicates completeness of sterilization, and they should be allowed to dry before handling. If stored, they should be marked with sterilization date.

Transporting of contaminated instruments

Reusable dental instruments that are to be reprocessed must be stored and transported safely in order to prevent cross contamination. These instruments include those classified as critical because they penetrate or touch open tissue (such as files, surgical burs, and scaler tips) as well as semicritical items that contact mucous membranes (such as rubber dam frames and mouth props). Procedure trays should be in the operatory, and contaminated instruments placed in the tray. During transport to the area set aside for cleaning, disinfecting, and sterilizing, the container should be covered and taken directly to the receiving area. If the instruments cannot be immediately processed, they are usually placed in a holding solution to prevent body fluids (blood, saliva) from drying on the instruments. Precleaning is a critical step prior to sterilization to removal all bioburden, which may interfere with the sterilization process.

Procedures for receiving items in or from dental laboratory

All items received and worked on in the dental laboratory are to be considered potentially infectious. There should be a specific receiving area for these items. It should be covered with impermeable paper and contain hand washing facilities and good ventilation. All articles received, generally prostheses or impressions, must be disinfected here before any other laboratory work is done. The technician should always wear personal protective equipment and use an EPA-registered intermediate- or high-level disinfectant. The disinfectant method is dependent on the type of material. If prostheses are heavily laden with calculus or adhesive, they can be precleaned before disinfection by placing them in a zippered plastic bag with disinfectant and using the ultrasonic cleaner. Completed prostheses are generally sent from the laboratory in containers containing mouth rinse. They must be disinfected again (at the chairside if possible) before use by rinsing them in tap water followed by a suitable disinfectant. If an impression cannot be immersed, it can be sprayed with disinfectant and wrapped in a saturated paper towel. Items that are heat-tolerant should be sterilized.

CDC categorization of patient care items

The Centers for Disease Control and Prevention (CDC) places patient care items into one of three categories in terms of how they must be processed after contamination. The first category is critical items, which are items that pierce soft tissue, touch bone, or come in contact with the bloodstream or normally sterile oral tissue. These include items such as scalers, blades, dental burs, and surgical instruments. The CDC mandates critical items must be cleaned and then sterilized using heat. Semicritical patient care items are those that come in contact with mucous membranes but do not penetrate them, or that come in contact with bone, the bloodstream, or normally sterile oral tissue. Semicritical items include things like the mouth mirror, reusable impression trays, and handpieces. They should be processed just like critical items, using cleaning followed by heat sterilization unless they are heat-sensitive. With heat-sensitive items, a high-level disinfectant can be used. Lastly, noncritical items are those that only come in contact with intact skin, such as a blood pressure cuff or stethoscope. These items should be cleaned and disinfected using a low-or intermediate-level disinfectant, depending on whether there is no or some visible blood on them.

Decontamination of instruments or operatory surfaces

Personal protective equipment should be worn during decontamination of instruments or operatory surfaces. Instruments should be decontaminated prior to servicing or shipment, with areas of inadequate decontamination clearly marked. Any surfaces including the operatory that are part of patient treatment should be covered with protective barriers which are changed between patients or cleaned and disinfected after each patient. Any reusable containers in contact with bodily fluids should also be cleaned and disinfected. There should be a written schedule for work area decontamination. The patient care room should not be carpeted or have cloth coverings anywhere. Its floors, walls and sinks should be cleaned regularly, and window treatments should be cleaned when perceptibly dusty or dirty.

Processing of instruments

There are seven steps involved in preparing contaminated instruments to be reused. They are as follows:

- Step 1 - brief holding or presoaking of the contaminated instruments in detergent, water, or enzyme solution to keep attached debris from drying
- Step 2 - precleaning to reduce the bioburden, surface microbial or organic material, before decontamination, generally through use of an ultrasonic cleaner
- Step 3 - corrosion control measures, drying and/or lubrication to moderate potential damage to the instrument
- Step 4 - packaging of the instruments to preserve sterility after sterilization
- Step 5 - sterilization or disinfection with a high-level agent to destroy all microorganisms present
- Step 6 - biological, chemical and/or mechanical monitoring of the sterilization process to ensure the sterilizer is performing properly
- Step 7 - correct handling of the processed instruments, including procedures like drying and cooling and proper techniques for storage, distribution, and opening of the instrument packages

Sterilization

Sterilization is a means of killing all microorganisms present. There are three methods of sterilization applicable to dentistry. These are sterilization using heat, gas, or liquid chemicals. Heat sterilization is performed in a steam sterilizer or autoclave at 250 to 375 °F. Gas sterilizers generally use ethylene oxide at a lower temperature of 72 to 140°F but for a longer time period; they are uncommon in dental settings. Articles that will not withstand heat are usually subjected to liquid chemical sterilization at room temperature. Liquid chemical sterilants, also classified as high-level disinfectants, include agents such as glutaraldehyde and hydrogen peroxide often in combination. Heat sterilization is the most effective method because if the sterilizer is working properly it can kill more resistant microorganisms such as *Mycobacterium* species as well as highly-resistant protein products such as bacterial endospores and fungal spores. The standard for biological monitoring of a sterilizer is whether it in fact can kill bacterial endospores. At present it is difficult to monitor effectiveness of liquid chemical sterilization.

Sterility assurance

Sterility assurance is the practice of measures to ensure that sterility of items processed through a sterilizer is achieved and maintained. These measures include suitable instrument packaging, the sterilization process, proper storage of sterilized packages, and use of monitoring procedures. A sterility assurance program can be instituted by selecting the correct procedure(s), developing a detailed written protocol for performance, including these protocols in employee training, and setting up biologic, chemical and mechanical monitoring systems of the performance. It is also advisable to set up a system of measuring results.

Precleaning contaminated instruments prior to sterilization

Most contaminated instruments are presoaked in water, detergent, or enzyme solution directly in the basket in which they will be precleaned. This step removes gross debris. The subsequent precleaning step reduces the bioburden of microbes and organic components. The FDA approves use of ultrasonic cleaners or instrument washers for precleaning. Manual scrubbing of instruments at this juncture is not recommended. Ultrasonic cleaners utilize ultrasonic energy, high frequency sound waves, to remove debris. Loose instruments are placed in removable cleaning baskets or cassette racks in the cleaner, covered, and cleaned per manufacturer's instructions. There should be enough cleaning solution to cover the instruments during the process. The cleaning time is variable depending on factors like the types of instruments being cleaned and what is on them; it usually varies from 4 to 16 minutes. Afterwards, the basket or cassette rack is taken out and rinsed with tap water. Cleaning solution should be drained or disposed of daily. In larger settings, FDA-regulated instrument washers are used for precleaning; they come in bench top, floor unit and large production versions. Utility gloves and personal protective equipment should always be worn.

Packaging instruments to be sterilized with dry heat or unsaturated chemicals

Instruments that are to be put in dry heat sterilizers can be wrapped in paper wrap, certain nylon plastic tubing, closed containers, wrappers made for perforated cassettes, or aluminum foil. Aluminum foil is not ideal as it can tear or be easily perforated, and if closed containers are used, a biological indicator must be included. Many plastic types of wrapping are unsuitable because they may char or melt. The appropriate types of wrapping for use with an unsaturated chemical sterilizer are paper wrap, paper and plastic peel pouches, and appropriately wrapped perforated cassettes. Closed containers cannot be used for chemical sterilization. Cloth wrapping is unsuitable as it absorbs chemical vapor, and certain plastics are also unsuitable as they can melt. Whatever sterilization process is to be used, the wrapping material must be FDA-approved.

Packaging instruments for heat sterilization

After presoaking, precleaning, and procedures such as drying to reduce instrument damage, the instruments are packaged for sterilization. All instrument packaging is regulated. Packaged instruments are medical devices and packaging must be FDA-approved. Instruments that are to be heat sterilized in a steam autoclave can be packaged in paper wrap and sealed with autoclave tape, placed within special nylon plastic tubing and heat sealed or taped, or put in self-sealing peel pouches with paper and plastic sides. If functional groups of instruments are being sterilized, the whole cassette can be wrapped. Heat sterilization precludes use of closed containers, cloth, and certain plastics. The envelope wrapping technique is often suggested if heavy paper is used. The instruments are placed in the center of the paper diagonal to the edges and an envelope is created by folding up the bottom, then each side, and finally a top flap followed by sealing with autoclave tape (a mechanical monitor). All packages should have some form of monitoring included (discussed further on another card).

Treatment of contaminated treatment tray in sterilization center

At the completion of a dental treatment and associated duties, the dental assistant brings the contaminated treatment tray into the sterilization center. Utility gloves, protective eyewear, and possibly a mask are worn while dealing with the contaminated treatment tray in this area. The contaminated instruments are submerged in a disinfecting holding solution if not sterilized immediately. Sharps and disposables should be properly discarded, including into biohazardous waste if appropriate. When ready to perform sterilization, the assistant first cleans the instruments in an ultrasonic cleaner for approximately 3 to 10 minutes, rinses, dries and bags them. The bagged instruments are tagged with indicator tape and placed into a sterilizer (usually steam under pressure). The high-speed handpiece should be rinsed with water or isopropyl alcohol and lubricated before bagging. The tray and many of the other items can simply be disinfected by the spray, wipe, spray again, and leave for 10 minutes rewipe method. The area is cleaned before removing the utility gloves, washing and the drying hands. When indicated, items in the sterilizer are removed with forceps (as they are hot).

Flash sterilization

Flash sterilization is the sterilization of unwrapped items at relative short exposure times. It is not recommended by the CDC for routine procedures but can be used in emergency situations requiring short turnaround times. For example, if the dentist drops a critical instrument but still needs it, flash sterilization might be done. When instruments are sterilized unwrapped, they must be handled aseptically afterwards at all points from removal from the sterilizer to patient care use. For example, sterile tongs and transport containers should be used. Procedures for flash sterilization and transport should be carefully outlined in writing, and monitoring practices should be in place.

Unsaturated chemical vapor sterilization of instruments

In unsaturated chemical vapor sterilization, a chemical solution with the active ingredient of 0.23% formaldehyde and other organic compounds is heated in a closed chamber along with the instruments. Once a temperature of about 270°F (132°C) and vaporization of the chemical solution is achieved during this heat-up cycle, the sterilizing cycle is initiated and maintained for 20 minutes. These phases are followed by a depressurization and an optional purge cycle. A drying phase is not needed because the chemical solution vaporizes. Another advantage of this method is that instruments will not corrode because the solution contains very little water. A disadvantage is that it is crucial to have adequate ventilation because of chemical vapor smells, which can be alleviated through use of a purge system.

Steam sterilizers

Steam sterilizers kill microorganisms by applying steam under pressure. High temperature is achieved quickly using steam. The three basic types of steam sterilizers or autoclaves are gravity displacement, vacuum pump (type B), and positive steam flush/pressure pulse. Each forces air out before generating steam. Mechanisms of air removal are via a drain for gravity displacement, a vacuum for type B, and repeated cycles of steam flushes and pressure pulses for the method by the same name. Standard sterilizing conditions are for 20 to 30 minutes once a steam temperature of 250°F (121.1°C) is achieved, but shorter times at a higher temperature of 273°F (134°C) are also used. Standard small office sterilizers usually have heat-up, sterilizing, depressurization, and drying cycles. Preset sterilizing cycles of 15 or 30 minutes at 250°F or 3 or 10 minutes at 273°F are commonly used. Wrapped packages should be inserted on their edge without stacking and unloaded only after drying to avoid wicking, the drawing in of external microbes. Flash sterilization (described elsewhere) should be done only in emergency situations for 3 to 10 minutes at 273°F. Hospital-type sterilizers are basically larger versions directly connected to a steam line.

Dry heat sterilization of instruments

Dry heat sterilizers heat air to kill microorganisms without generation of steam. This necessitates higher temperatures than other sterilization methods. The biggest advantage of dry heat sterilizers is that they do not corrode instruments. Static air or oven-type dry heat sterilizers have heating coils that generate heat inside through natural convection which is then transmitted to the instruments. Once an internal temperature of 320°F (160°C) is achieved, this temperature is maintained for 1 to 2 hours for sterilization. Other dry heat sterilizers use forced air circulation or rapid heat transfer. These sterilizers begin their sterilization cycle once 375°F or 190°C is attained. Wrapped or unwrapped instruments should be kept at this temperature for 12 or 6 minutes respectively. Whichever type is utilized, the chamber door must remain closed throughout sterilization to maintain the desired temperature. Timing outlines should be adhered to, and routine spore testing with *Bacillus atrophaeus* is essential.

Less common sterilization methods

Ethylene oxide gas will kill microorganisms at low temperatures (~120°F) and is useful for sterilizing plastic and rubber items. Its drawbacks are long sterilization times (up to 12 hours), the need for lengthy post-sterilization aeration to get rid of gas molecules, and potential toxicity. Wet items cannot be sterilized with this method. A new but expensive technique that also uses low temperatures utilizes vaporized hydrogen peroxide gas plasma. So-called "bead sterilizers" have been used in the past but are not often recommended, as they are difficult to monitor and deal with aseptically. This type of sterilization involves glass beads heated to about 450°F. Instruments to be sterilized are briefly plunged into the glass beads. Hot mineral oil baths are another antiquated and unacceptable method of sterilization.

Sterilizing heat-labile items

Heat-labile items that do not penetrate tissue (such as rubber dam frames and x-ray collimators) must be sterilized using a liquid sterilant/high-level disinfectant. For example, 2 to 3.4% glutaraldehyde or 7% hydrogen peroxide may be used as a sterilant/disinfectant. Gloves and other protective equipment should be worn throughout involved procedures. Sterilant solutions often have to be prepared as indicated by the manufacturer before use and may have a restricted life. These solutions should be clearly marked with chemical name, date, and other useful information and kept in a covered container. They should also be tested for concentration periodically using a chemical test kit and replaced if necessary. The items to be sterilized should be precleaned, rinsed, and dried initially. Then they are placed into the liquid sterilant using a perforated tray or tongs, taking care that they are completely immersed in the solution. The appropriate immersion time should be indicated on the product label. Using aseptic technique (usually sterile tongs), the sterilized items are rinsed with sterile water, dried, and placed in a sterile container until use.

Sterilization failure

Sterilization failure is an extremely rare occurrence if sterilization is performed correctly. Sterilization failure can be due to improper precleaning or packaging of the instruments, use of an unacceptable method of sterilization, or improper loading, timing or temperature setting related to the sterilization process. Instruments that are not precleaned properly can still have attached debris that prevents contact between the item and the sterilizing agent. If the wrong packaging material is used, the sterilizing agent might be prevented from contact with the contaminated item or the packaging material might melt. Contact with the sterilizing agent can also be retarded if too much packaging or a closed container is used. Cloth wraps are unacceptable in chemical vapor sterilizers as they absorb chemicals. Method problems are generally related to use of sterilization for heat-sensitive items like plastic or attempts to use chemical vapors or dry heat to sterilize things in solution or water. Overloading or failing to separate packages can impede penetration of the sterilizing agent. Insufficient heat or sterilization time will not kill all microorganisms and/or spores.

Proper handling of instrument packages after sterilization

Instrument packages that have been sterilized must be dried and cooled before use. Most steam sterilizers have some type of incorporated drying cycle, and unsaturated chemical vapor and dry heat sterilizers generate packages that are dry at the end. The drying prevents wicking, the drawing in of microbes through wet wrapping. The packages will be warm and should be cooled gradually. Sterile packages should be stored in enclosed cabinets in dry, relatively low dust areas and away from water sources. Instruments sterilized in FDA-approved packaging should be sterile at least 6 months if stored properly but a shorter turnaround time is suggested. Instruments flash sterilized unwrapped have no storage life. It is suggested that sterile instrument packages be stored away from the patient care area and transmitted to and opened at the chairside when they are needed. Packages should be checked for intactness before opening. They should be opened with clean, ungloved hands after seating the patient. If rearrangement of instruments is needed at that point, sterile tongs should be used.

Protecting dental instruments for reuse

One of the biggest concerns regarding protection of dental instruments is prevention of corrosion. Stainless steel instruments do not corrode significantly when in contact with moisture and heat, but those containing carbon steel do have this problem. Measures to reduce corrosion include cleaning as promptly as possible, avoiding long storage in water or chloride solutions, use of cleaning solutions specifically designed for cleaning the instruments, and adequate rinsing after cleaning. There are rust inhibitors available that can be used on carbon steel instruments before steam sterilization, and alternatively they can be processed using a dry heat or unsaturated chemical vapor sterilizer. For the latter methods, drying the items prior to sterilization also retards corrosion. A general protection method is the avoidance of contact between various instruments during cleaning.

Monitoring Equipment and Sterilizers

Biological monitoring

Since it is impossible to directly test each piece of sterilized equipment for effectiveness of sterilization, the process must be monitored by biologic, chemical, and/or mechanical monitoring. Biological monitoring, also termed spore testing, basically involves putting very resistant bacteria spores into the system and later checking to see whether they have been killed. The biological indicators (BIs) generally used are strips (or vials for steam sterilization) of spores of *Geobacillus stearothermophilus* for steam autoclaves and unsaturated chemical vapor chambers, and *Bacillus atrophaeus* spore strips in dry heat or ethylene oxide sterilizers. After each sterilization, the BIs are removed aseptically and incubated in culture medium for 2 to 7 days at 55°F for *G. stearothermophilus* or 37°F for *B. atrophaeus*. The growth medium will turn cloudy or change color if spores are present. Vial-type indicators are squeezed or have caps that are pushed down to break an internal ampule and subsequently incubated at 55°F. Spore testing should be performed minimally once a week. A control strip or vial that was not put in the sterilizer should be cultured similarly for reference.

Complete sterilization monitoring program

The CDC advocates that dental offices include as part of a complete sterilization monitoring program a chemical indicator on the inside of every package. If the internal chemical indicator is not visible, an external chemical indicator should be placed as well on every package to be processed. Every cycle should also undergo mechanical monitoring, which entails observation of all gauges, displays, and readouts. In addition, biologic monitoring in the form of spore testing appropriate for the type of sterilizer utilized should be carried out at least weekly. Documentation of each type of monitoring is essential for sterility assurance and should be kept in case problems are identified.

Aluminum foil test

The aluminum foil test is a method of evaluating the functionality of an ultrasonic cleaning unit. A piece of aluminum foil about 1 inch shorter than the length of the chamber by about 1 inch longer than its depth is cut. The foil is dipped vertically into the chamber filled with solution without touching the bottom. The unit is turned on for 20 seconds. The foil is taken out and scrutinized for pebbling or small indentations on the foil. If the ultrasonic unit is operating properly, this pebbling will be uniformly found on the previously submerged portion of the foil. If there are areas with no pebbling, the unit may need to be serviced.

Spore testing of small office sterilizers

Appropriate times for testing

Biological monitoring or spore testing of small office sterilizers used in a dental office can be done in-house or through a mail-in monitoring service. In-office monitoring is more cumbersome and requires purchase of a number of supplies. Spore testing should be done once a week to confirm that the sterilizer is functioning and being used properly. It should also be performed anytime a new type of packaging material or tray is employed to make sure the sterilizing agent is contacting the surface of instruments. It is also appropriate when initiating use of a new sterilizer for familiarization purposes and initially after a device is repaired to make sure it is functioning correctly. If some change is instituted in the sterilizing procedure, spore testing should be done. Biological monitoring should be done every time sterilization is used for implantable devices to ensure that microorganisms are not implanted; in this case the device should not be installed until results are known. Lastly, spore testing should be done after sterilization runs done by employees undergoing training to make sure they are doing them properly.

Process

The appropriate biological indicator should be inserted into a suitable type of wrapping, placed into the center of a load to be processed in the sterilizer, and treated in exactly the same manner as contaminated instruments in the sterilizing process. The package containing the biological indicator should be clearly marked if necessary, and if a spore strip is utilized, it should not be removed from its blue envelope. The center of the load is usually appropriate for the BI as that is the most difficult area for the sterilization to reach. After processing, the test date, sterilizer type, time and temperature used, type of monitor, and operator should be documented. The biological indicator is removed from the sterilizer. It and an unprocessed control indicator are sent to the sterilization monitoring service or incubated and observed for spores in-house to make certain of test reliability and sterilization success. Monitoring results should be recorded and maintained. If a sterilization failure is indicated, the sterilizer must be removed from service and spore testing done under controlled conditions.

Chemical monitoring of sterilization process

Chemical monitors are indicators that change color or transform physically during the sterilization process. Externally-applied autoclave tape and special markings on certain pouches and bags are examples of chemical monitors that change color once a certain high temperature has been reached. Autoclave tape develops dark stripes and other types of chemical monitors have distinct color changes within a certain region. There are also chemical monitors called integrated indicators that are designed to be put inside every wrapped instrument package, where they undergo color changes during sterilization. If these internal indicators are not visible, an external chemical monitor such as autoclave tape should also be applied. After the sterilization process, if external chemical monitors have not changed color indicating a sterilization failure, the processed instruments should not be used and spore testing should be done. Processed instruments should also not be used if after opening it is clear that an internal chemical monitor has not changed color. When internal indicators have not changed color, either no sterilization was performed or the sterilizing agent did not get through the packaging for some reason.

Follow-up procedures in event of sterilization failure

The first step in the event of a sterilization failure is the removal of that sterilizer from service and complete re-processing of any instruments sterilized since the previous spore test. Sterilization procedures then need to be scrutinized. This involves review of all chemical monitoring records since the most recent negative spore test. Loading and operating methods should be reviewed to determine if any changes had been made, if anything had been done differently during the failed cycle, or whether new personnel were involved. Any problems identified should be addressed and the sterilizer retested afterwards using the same conditions as during the sterilization failure. All 3 types of monitoring should be included during this cycle and all gauges and readouts should be observed during the process. If biologic and chemical monitoring tests are negative, the sterilizer can be returned to service at this point, but if the spore test is positive the machine must be repaired or replaced. Later a new or repaired sterilizer must be spore tested three times with negative results before any instruments can be sterilized in it.

Occupational Safety/Administrative Procedures

Occupational Safety

Improving negative environmental impact of infection control procedures in dental office

Almost all aspects of infection control in the dental office can be made more eco-friendly and improve upon the generally negative environmental impact they generate. The sterilization process, for example, can be made more eco-friendly by using a large instrument washer to clean multiple cassettes instead of an ultrasonic cleaner over and over, cutting down water and chemical use. Some personal protective equipment can be washed and reused instead of being disposed of. The vast majority of waste is not regulated medical waste and can be flushed down the sink. Use of disinfectant wipes instead of saturated paper towels cuts down on waste. Digital radiography eliminates the need for developer and fixer chemicals used with traditional radiography. Paper use can be diminished through use of digital patient records. These are just some examples of eco-friendly measures

Tenets of infection control

The World Health Organization developed three basic tenets of infection control in 2003 in reaction to the SARS or severe acute respiratory syndrome epidemic ensuing at that time. Many now believe that there should be a fourth tenet as well. The first three are to protect the patient, the practitioner, and repeat both if necessary. The newest tenet is to protect the environment. It is not enough just to protect the patient in situations where infections can be spread. It is equally as important to safeguard the health care worker and to practice measures if possible that will not generate excess waste, bring in potentially dangerous chemicals, or cause adverse tissue reactions.

Elements of exposure control plan

An exposure control plan evaluates the exposure risk of each employee according to the person's duties and establishes safety measures to prevent exposure. These measures may include the use of safety-engineered devices, such as syringes with retractable needles. The plan must also outline the types of personal protective equipment necessary for different procedures and types of possible exposure. The plan should include measures to minimize exposure to blood and body fluids. Additionally, the plan must address protocols for post-exposure prophylaxis for occupational exposure to bloodborne pathogens, including any necessary follow-up monitoring or treatment, the name of the person responsible for directing the care of the individual, the place where testing will be carried out, and the information necessary to ensure adequate assessment of the exposure. The exposure control plan should also include tuberculosis control measures, such as TB screening, and should address the issue of pregnancy and exposures that may pose a risk to the pregnancy or the developing fetus.

Breach of infection control

According to the CDC, the steps for assessing a breach of infection control include:

- Identifying the type of breach: Determine how the breach occurred and what risk of exposure exists. Take corrective action as soon as possible to prevent further breaches and review techniques.
- Gathering additional data: Determine when breach occurred and who was exposed, and carry out a literature review and/or consult with experts.

- Notifying key stakeholders: These may include infection control professionals, health departments, government agencies, accreditation agencies, risk management, and all those who risk exposure.
- Assessing the breach: Classify as category A breach (gross error with high risk of exposure) or category B (lesser risk of exposure).
- Making a decision about patient testing/notification: Classify as category A if notification and testing necessary or category B if the need to notify is balanced against low risk.
- Communicating: Materials to communicate are developed.
- Post-exposure prophylaxis: Outline logistical matters—who, where, when, how.
- Media and legal issues: Make media announcement if indicated and consult legal representatives for liability issues.

Sterilization logs and training records

Sterilization logs may vary somewhat but are used to monitor sterilization and provide evidence that the process was carried out correctly. Elements of a log often include the date, the identification number of the item, the contents, the beginning and ending times or the duration, the temperature, the pressure (PSI), the results of the chemical indicator, the spore count, and the signature of the person responsible. These records may be reviewed when sterilization fails in order to try to determine the cause or when products are recalled. The log and dating of the sterilized items also helps to ensure proper rotation of supplies.

Training records provide documented evidence that infection control training was carried out, the type of training, and the participants. Dental health care personnel should receive training regarding infection control principle, employment-associated risk factors, preventive measures, and post-exposure protocols. Training should be appropriate for the individual's duties and responsibilities.

Workplace safety and health standards development

The Occupational Safety and Health Administration creates advisory committees to evaluate standards that it or other organizations deem important (such as federal or state agencies or the National Institute for Occupational Safety and Health). If OSHA decides to initiate, change or get rid of a standard, it circulates its intention to do so in the Federal Register. The public is given a time period to respond to or provide additional information regarding the proposed new rules as well as notification regarding related hearings. New standards including related clarifications and rationale (or if appropriate notice of no change) are also published ultimately in the Federal Register. If circumstances arise that OSHA deems critical and uncovered by present standards, it can issue a binding emergency temporary standard until it has been reviewed as above.

Standards and Protocols

OSHA

OSHA, the Occupational Safety and Health Administration, was established in 1971 subsequent to the federal Occupational Safety and Health Act of 1970. OSHA's mission is the promotion of workplace safety and health through compelling enforcement measures, assistance with outreach and compliance, and affiliations and cooperative programs. OSHA provides a number of functions to these ends. These functions include promotion of workplace safety programs, research, outlining responsibilities and rights of workers and employers, acting as a repository for recordkeeping regarding injuries and illnesses, developing training programs, spelling out standards for health and safety, and working with state agencies. Twenty-four states plus two U. S. territories have OSHA-approved programs. OSHA has established standards for a multitude of workplace hazards, including but not limited to hazardous waste, infectious diseases, and toxic substances. Employers are expected to achieve these standards by any combination of acceptable stated means. OSHA also covers circumstances not specifically covered elsewhere in the OSHA General Duty Clause.

Goals of the OSHA 2003-2008 Strategic Management Plan

The overall objective of the OSHA 2003-2008 Strategic Management Plan has been the reduction of deaths, illnesses, and injuries in the workplace. OSHA's goals are in support of the Department of Labor's Strategic Plan and its goals which are a prepared and secure workforce and quality workplaces. OSHA broke down its Strategic Management Plan into three underlying goals. They are: (1) reduction in occupational hazards through direct intervention such as training programs and workplace inspections, (2) promotion of a culture of safety and health within the workplace by means such as compliance assistance and cooperative programs, and (3) maximization of effectiveness and efficiency by furthering the capabilities of employees and strengthening infrastructure. OSHA defined specific percentage improvements desired in a number of different areas, for example the reduction of workplace fatalities over the 5 year period by 15% and illnesses and injuries by 20%.

Relationship between OSHA and state safety and health programs

States can and are encouraged by OSHA to work out and enforce their own job safety and health programs. OSHA will fund up to 50% of the working costs of state programs that have been endorsed under the Occupational Safety and Health Act. These state programs must be at least as comprehensive as the federal standards to receive endorsement and funds. State programs may encompass only public sector employees or they may also incorporate private sector workers. All but three of the 26 states with current OSHA plans cover both the public and private sectors. Federal employees still fall under the umbrella of federal OSHA regulations.

Complaints related to workplace safety and health hazards

Safety or health hazards occurring at a worksite or by an employee can be reported by anyone to OSHA. The complainant can request that his or her name be withheld from the employer. Complaints can be filed online at www.osha.gov using form OSHA-7 or by printing out the form, completing it, and then faxing or mailing it to the OSHA Regional Office. Employees who have been discriminated against for exercising their rights or refusing to work under unsafe conditions as outlined by OSHA can file discrimination complaints with the OSHA Regional Office. Then OSHA will stage no inquiry, conduct an inquiry, or perform an onsite inspection of the hazards listed in the complaint. If OSHA decides to conduct an onsite inspection, it is generally done without warning to the employer, who may request a warrant necessitating a return visit. The OSHA inspectors typically hold an explanatory opening conference at the site, carry out a walk-through inspection looking for hazards, and afterwards hold a closing conference at which they discuss hazards observed and possible citations and distribute a copy of *Employer Rights and Responsibilities Following an OSHA Inspection*. An employee representative is present throughout.

Inspections performed by OSHA

OSHA, the Occupation Safety and Health Administration, performs 5 types of inspections, listed below in order of decreasing priority. They are investigations of the following:

1. Imminent danger, situations that could result in death or grave physical harm
2. Catastrophes and fatal accidents, circumstances that resulted in death or hospitalization of at least three employees
3. Complaints and referrals, situations in which employees have made official complaints or anyone else has contacted authorities about unsafe or unhealthy conditions in a workplace
4. Programmed inspections, periodic evaluations at sites identified by OSHA as potentially highly hazardous
5. Follow-up inspections, evaluations done to determine whether an employer has rectified prior violations

OSHA standards eliciting the most inspections and/or citations in dental offices and laboratories

By far, the two OSHA standards eliciting the most inspections and/or violation citations in dental office and laboratories are the OSHA Bloodborne Pathogens Standard followed by the OSHA Hazard Communication Standard. These are the most often cited in both the Offices and Clinics of Dentists Industry Group and the Medical and Dental Laboratories Industry Group. Over $35,000 worth of penalties were assessed by OSHA for violations by dental offices or laboratories of the Bloodborne Pathogens Standard between for the 12-month period of October 2006 to September 2007. Other types of citations include violations related to sanitation, exit routes, electrical wiring, etc.

Potential outcomes of OSHA inspections

The OSHA inspector will report his or her observations to the area director who makes a determination regarding violations. OSHA then issues citations to the employer for violations. The employer has 15 days to dispute the terms using the *Notice of Intent to Contest*, sent to the OSHA Review Commission. Violations generally involve some sort of financial penalty issued along with the citation or shortly thereafter. Violations fall into one of six categories. They are considered "willful" if the employer knew of the hazard but made no attempt to eliminate it, "serious" if the danger has potential to cause death or serious physical harm but the employer was unaware of the violation, and "other-than-serious" if the hazard would not cause death or serious illness. Violations can also be classified as "de minimis" or not directly affecting health or safety, "failure to abate" referring to violations previously cited and not dealt with, or "repeated" where the same type of violation recurs over repeated visits.

Exposure control plan and other written documents

OSHA mandates that a written exposure control plan be developed and available to all appropriate employees. The exposure control plan should include the following: information about how exposure is determined; the schedules and procedures for compliance, hepatitis B vaccinations, evaluation of exposure episodes, postexposure medical assessment and follow-up; and methods for communication of biohazards. The plan should contain any recordke*eping concerning the OSHA Bloodborne Pathogens Standard. It should also include information about new safety devices, and the plan should be revised yearly or when new laws, techniques or equipment become available. There should also be a written CDC-compliant tuberculosis infection control plan. In addition, there should be written policies, procedures and records related to health of individual personnel including such features as immunizations received, medical conditions, training, work restrictions, and latex allergies if present.

Developing patient trust regarding office infection control procedures

First of all, there should be clear-cut established infection control procedures in the dental office. Employees should be knowledgeable about these procedures. They can give patients written information about the procedures, offer patients tours of the workplace including the sterilizing room, and generally maintain a clean and dust-free environment. Furthermore, the dental worker can directly show the patient that he/she is practicing infection control by making sure the patient sees the dental worker washing his or her hands, putting on new gloves, and unpacking sterile instruments from their sterilizing packages

Office safety coordinator

Every dental office should have a safety officer, who is generally a dental assistant or hygienist. He or she is responsible for systematizing and supervising office safety and maintaining all related documents. The officer is responsible for tasks such as the following: preparing, reviewing, and revising all procedural manuals and control plans (especially infection control and hazardous materials); training of personnel; monitoring compliance with safety procedures; overseeing hepatitis B vaccination programs; and assessment of exposure incidents. Many of the safety officer's duties are related to overseeing equipment safety, such as spore testing for sterilizers, proper disposal of regulated medical waste, keeping smoke alarms in operating order, and maintaining certification of radiographic equipment.

<u>Office safety documents and records maintained by office safety coordinator</u>

Office safety documents and records fall into three categories. There are regulatory documents that should be available, including the Occupational Safety and Health Administration's (OSHA) Bloodborne Pathogens and Hazard Communications Standards plus state and local regulations. Next there are policy documents, which include written infection exposure control and hazard communication programs for the office, CDC-compliant tuberculosis infection control and personal health plans, and action plans for fires or other emergencies. Safety procedures not encompassed by OSHA standards, such as instrument sterilization, should be included as well. The OSHA poster entitled "Job Safety and Health Protection", which should be posted, is considered a policy document. Lastly, there are a whole range of records that should be kept including but not limited to training records related to bloodborne pathogens and hazards, employee medical records, spore testing, radiographic equipment certification, cataloging of hazardous chemicals, and safety data sheets.

Office staff training as part of infection control program

OSHA requires that office staff members who might be exposed to infections be trained about infection control when they are first employed and, thereafter, at least annually. The instructor must be conversant about the subjects covered and the dental office setting and should welcome questions during the presentation. The training should include a thorough explanation of causes, signs, epidemiology, transmission and prevention of bloodborne illnesses and tuberculosis. It should also include a rundown of the office's exposure control plan, information about the equipment and supplies that aid in reduction of transmission, facts regarding the offered hepatitis B vaccination, procedures related to exposure incidents, and explanations about biohazard designations and color coding. The audience should be given and made aware of the OSHA Bloodborne Pathogens Standards and other pertinent infection control laws.

Occupational exposure, postexposure medical evaluation, and follow-up

All occupational exposures to potentially infectious materials such as blood or saliva should be documented and reported. A medical evaluation and follow-up must be offered free of charge to the employee by a licensed physician or nurse practitioner in an office where the OSHA Bloodborne Pathogens Standard is available. The physician must counsel the employee about the results and possible scenarios and send a written confirmation to the employer that such events have occurred. In addition, if patients can be identified as the source of transmission, they should be asked to be tested for their hepatitis B and HIV status. Exposure incidents should be reviewed afterwards to glean out they might be prevented in the future.

OSHA Bloodborne Pathogens Standard

The Occupational Safety and Health Administration Bloodborne Pathogens Standard covers protection measures for exposure to blood and other potentially infectious materials (OPIMS). It states that every facility where such exposure might occur, such as the dental office, must review the standard. The facility must also prepare a written exposure control plan including how it plans to protect and train workers. It must make available appropriate biohazard communications via training and use of signs and labels. Workers must be offered the hepatitis B vaccination series as well as medical evaluations and follow-ups if they are exposed. Medical and training records must be maintained for each employee. Standard precautions must be followed in the facility with respect to blood, all bodily fluids except sweat, nonintact skin, and mucous membranes. This includes both engineering and work practice controls such as use of hand washing and handling of contaminated sharps as well as use and disposal of personal protective equipment. The Standard also covers appropriate housekeeping procedures, management of regulated waste, and procedures for contaminated laundry. It does not address instrument sterilization.

Regulations governing infection control in dental offices

The main regulations are dictated by OSHA, the Occupational Safety and Health Administration, which is part of the U. S. Department of Labor. OSHA has set up a blood-borne pathogens standard as well as another for protection against hazardous chemicals. These standards must be followed in every state and are monitored. Twenty-six states have OSHA divisions within their state departments of labor. Additional state and local regulations vary regarding dental office infection control, and most are concerned with medical waste management, instrument sterilization and spore testing. The Food and Drug Administration (FDA), a division of the U. S. Department of Health and Human Services, also affects infection control because it regulates production and labeling of medical devices (of which there are many used in the dental office), antimicrobial handwashing solutions, and mouth rinses. The Environmental Protection Agency (EPA) is also involved in infection control as it regulates medical waste and provides guidelines for disinfectants.

Categories of possible occupational exposure

There are three categories of possible occupational exposure as pertaining to the OSHA Bloodborne Pathogens Standard. They are based on the type of tasks performed and the risk of exposure to blood and other potentially infectious materials (OPIMS). Category 1 applies to all jobs that directly involve exposure to blood and OPIMS; the dentist, dental assistants, hygienists, and dental laboratory technicians fall into this category. Category 2 applies to tasks that generally do not involve blood or OPIM exposure but may occasionally perform unplanned Category 1 chores such as those performed by the receptionist or coordinator. Category 3 tasks are devoid of blood or OPIM exposure, such as those of the bookkeeper or insurance handler.

Exposure control plan

The OSHA Bloodborne Pathogens Standard mandates that facilities to which it applies develop a written exposure control plan. There are 4 major areas that it should include. The first is determination of the probability and types of occupational exposure that might occur to any employee in the office. The employer also must make of schedule of how and when each of the stipulations in the Standard will be implemented. The plan should include a means of evaluating the circumstances surrounding exposure incidents in terms of things such as source patient, protective equipment used, and route of exposure. It should also describe the safety devices to be utilized for prevention of sharps injuries, how they are to be evaluated, and why certain ones are selected.

Minimal requirements for compliance with biohazards communication section of OSHA Bloodborne Pathogens Standard

Employers are required to provide an available copy of the standard and free training to any employee with possible occupational exposure. The minimum requirements for this training should include explanations of epidemiology and symptoms of bloodborne diseases, modes of their transmission, an outline of the exposure control plan, and how to recognize means of exposure. The training should also cover ways to prevent and reduce exposure, including engineering controls, work practices, and personal protective equipment. The employees should be informed about the availability of and need for hepatitis B vaccination and post-exposure procedures and evaluations. Biohazards communication should also involve use and clarification of required signs and labels.

OSHA-required procedures for post-exposure medical evaluation and follow-up

When there is a potentially infectious exposure incident, it is the responsibility of the employer to send the exposed employee to a healthcare professional for testing for hepatitis B virus (HBV) and human immunodeficiency virus (HIV). The only exceptions would be if the employee does not consent or if the employee's viral status to the above agents is already known. Consenting employees are tested and given their results along with an evaluation as to appropriate course of action by the healthcare professional. The healthcare professional should be provided with an incident report, HBV vaccination status, and other pertinent information by the employer before testing. In turn, the health care professional is required to give the employer a post-evaluation written opinion, which indicates that the employee was informed of results and whether other measures are indicated. This written opinion should be kept confidentially in the employee's medical file.

Hepatitis B vaccination

Hepatitis B transmission is one of the greatest concerns in healthcare settings and there are effective vaccines for the disease. The OSHA standard addresses this issue. It requires the employer to provide a copy of the standard to each healthcare professional, vaccine-related training, and the option for a free series of the hepatitis B vaccine within 10 days of employment. An employee can either accept or decline the offer for vaccination. If the employee accepts, the vaccine must be administered by a licensed physician or other appropriate healthcare profession (for example, a nurse practitioner). If the employee declines, he/she must sign a declination statement. If, at a later time, the employee wishes to be vaccinated, the employer must provide vaccination free of charge. The healthcare professional evaluates each employee for vaccination, previous protection, or contraindications to vaccination. The health care professional performs the vaccinations and provides a written evaluation to the employee. One copy is to be maintained in the employee's confidential medical file.

Employee's records

Both medical and training records should be included in an employee's file. The OSHA Bloodborne Pathogens Standard indicates that training records should be kept for at least 3 years and includes the dates of training, the topics that were covered, the names and qualifications of the instructors, and the names and job titles of all present. Medical records must be kept longer, at least 30 years after termination of employment. They must include the employee's name and Social Security number, the employee's hepatitis B vaccination status and all associated documentation, and any occupational exposure incidents including the healthcare professional's post-exposure written opinion.

OSHA-required engineering and work practice controls

The OSHA Bloodborne Pathogens Standard mandates a number of engineering and work practice controls to minimize exposure to infectious agents. An engineering control is something that can impact the hazard itself such as use of puncture-resistant sharps containers or retractable scalpels. For example, both disposable and reusable contaminated sharps should be placed directly into sharps containers (the latter for later processing). Work practice controls are measures taken during a task that reduce the likelihood of exposure. These include things such as thorough handwashing practices after removal of gloves or personal protective equipment, flushing of mucous membranes if exposed, minimizing spatter of blood or saliva (for example with use of a rubber dam and/or evacuation), and limiting activities such as drinking and eating in the work area.

PPE

The OSHA Bloodborne Pathogens Standard states that an employer must provide free of charge personal protective equipment (PPE) to employees with the potential for occupational exposure. The employer must also make sure that the employee uses the PPE, that a range of suitable sizes is available in the office, that provisions are made for cleaning and/or disposal of PPE, and that it will be repaired or replaced to preserve effectiveness if necessary. PPE falls into several categories. The first category is gloves, which should be donned any time the employee may be in contact with blood, saliva, mucous membranes, broken skin, or contaminated surfaces. The next type of personal protective equipment is anything that shields the face. This category of PPE includes masks covering the nose and mouth and protective eyewear, such as goggles or glasses. Protective clothing must be worn as an outer garment to protect against exposure, taken off afterwards, and laundered at the office or by a service. The type of protective clothing (for example lab coats, aprons, gowns, etc.) depends on expected exposure. PPE penetrated by blood or saliva should be replace immediately.

Hazardous chemicals

A hazardous chemical is one that presents either a physical or health hazard. A physical hazard is any chemical for which there is scientific verification that it is unstable in some way. This can mean it is a combustible liquid, a compressed gas, unstable or water reactive, flammable, explosive, can ignite spontaneously, or is an organic peroxide and oxidizer. Basically physical hazards fall into two categories, those that are flammable and those that are reactive. Flammable chemicals are those that can quickly or thoroughly vaporize at atmospheric pressure and room temperature or that burn easily. Reactive or unstable chemicals are those that are susceptible to release of energy, including ones that are normally unstable chemically but do not explode or materials that are reactive with water. A health hazard is any material that can cause major health damage or death quickly despite prompt medical attention. Health hazards must have warning labels indicating the specific health hazard, including the target organ affected.

OSHA Hazard Communication Standard

Hazard communication ranks second in number of citations issued by the Occupational Safety and Health Administration in dental settings. The OSHA Hazard Communication Standard (also known as the HazCom Standard and the "Employee Right to Know") applies to any workplace setting in which chemicals are used. The Standard is designed to prevent employee exposures to hazardous chemicals. It mandates that chemical manufacturers evaluate and provide information to employers (who must in turn convey this to employees) about the hazards associated with their chemicals. It is comprehensive meaning it covers all hazardous chemicals that might be encountered in a variety of workplaces while excluding things generally for private consumption such as drugs, tobacco, alcohol, and consumer products. The scope of the HazCom standard includes setting up a written HazCom Program (WHCP) in affected workplaces, provision of Safety Data Sheets (SDS) by the manufacturer, use of special protective equipment when using hazardous chemicals, and engineering and workplace controls.

NFPA's method of labeling chemicals

The National Fire Protection Association (NFPA) suggests chemical labels colored as follows: red for fire hazards, yellow for reactivity, and blue for health hazards. Containers for chemicals are often labeled with a diamond-shaped area on the front with 4 subdivisions. At the apex is a red fire hazard classification with numbering system as follows: 0 for non-combustible; 1 and 2 for caution for combustible when heated or a combustible liquid; 3 for a flammable liquid; and 4 for danger due to a flammable gas or very flammable liquid. Below the red diamond are blue and yellow ones for health and reactivity hazards respectively. For blue health hazards, the numbering system is as follows: 0 for no unusual hazard; 1 for possible irritation; 2 and 3 for harmful if inhaled and corrosive or toxic respectively; and 4 for danger and the possibility of fatality. For yellow reactivity ratings, the numbering system is as follows: 0 for stable; 1 for caution of possible reactivity if heated or mixed with water; 2 for instability under the same conditions, 3 for dangerous around sparks or heating under confinement; and 4 for explosive at room temperature. The label has a white diamond on the bottom indicating appropriate personal protective equipment (designated A to G).

Developing a workplace written hazard communication program

Workplaces utilizing hazardous chemicals (including dental offices) are required under the OSHA Hazard Communication Standard to develop a custom-made written hazard communication program (WHCP) for compliance. Initially copies of the HazCom Standard should be given to each employee for familiarization. A HazCom compliance officer and a backup officer (generally the dentist) should be internally identified. A list should be compiled of all the chemicals used or manufactured at the workplace including their locations. Methods for use of hazardous chemicals in situations like performance of nonroutine tasks or while employing part-time or contract workers should be described in the WHCP. Methods of labeling containers should be clearly defined. Safety Data Sheets (SDSs) should be obtained for each hazardous chemical and maintained in an organized manner. A training coordinator should be named and details of a training program regarding the HazCom described. In addition, if chemical formulas are trade secrets the manufacturer or supplier still has the responsibility of indicating the appropriate protective measures which should be included in the WHCP.

Safety Data Sheets

Safety Data Sheets (SDSs) are information sheets that must be conveyed by chemical manufacturers and importers with any product containing hazardous chemicals. Official SDS forms are issued by the U. S. Department of Labor and OSHA for compliance with the OSHA Hazard Communication Standard. They should be kept in a central organized location as well as available near where the chemical is used. There are 16 sections on a SDS which contain information about the manufacturer, the hazardous ingredients in the preparation and identity information (including the NFPA Hazard rating), the physical and chemical characteristics of the chemical, fire and explosion hazard data, reactivity data, health hazard data, applicable precautions for safe handling and use, any additional information, and control measures (such as personal protective equipment) required. Other SDS sections also have information regarding special precautions required and/or emergency and first aid procedures.

Chemical inventory form and hazardous chemical labels

A chemical inventory form should include the inventory date and name of the dental office. Each chemical that is utilized in the office should be listed by its chemical name. The hazard classification from 0 to 4 should be listed for each possible distinction as a health hazard, fire hazard, or a possible reactivity. For each chemical, the appropriate personal protective equipment to use should also be listed, the physical state (for example gas, liquid or solid) should be indicated, and the manufacturer should be recorded. It is helpful to leave space for comments as well. A challenge in the dental office is the fact that hazardous chemicals may be part of dental materials kits without proper labeling making it difficult to correctly inventory them. Not all manufacturers follow the National Fire Protection Association labeling recommendations (described on another card). The minimum requirements according to the HazCom Standard regarding labeling of hazardous chemicals are inclusion of the identity of the hazardous chemical(s), the appropriate hazard warning including target organs if a health hazard, and information about the manufacturer or other responsible party.

Determining hazardous chemical problems in the office

Employees often feel that there may be a problem regarding hazardous chemicals in the office. For example, they are getting headaches or dermatitis. The first step should be to actually ascertain whether there is a problem. Some problems can be detected through use of monitoring equipment, for example badges or air samplers that undergo color changes in the presence of certain chemicals. The employer may need to seek advice from authorities such as an industrial hygienist or health or air quality departments. If there appears to be an issue, engineering controls, work practice controls, and/or personal protective equipment (PPE) can be changed to potentially eliminate the problem. Engineering controls (the most effective) are any procedures or materials that can reduce hazardous chemical exposure, for example use of sterilization rather than glutaraldehyde. Work practice controls are any procedural changes that can diminish the likelihood of exposure, for example, use of a fume hood for ventilation. Alterations in PPE use are generally the least effective means of dealing with these issues.

Essential components of training regarding the HazCom Standard

Any employee who might come in contact with hazardous chemicals, even non-routinely, must be trained regarding the OSHA Hazardous Communication Standard (HazCom). This training must occur at the time of employment, every time a new hazard is presented, and once a year for all continuing employees. Training can be done by the designated HazCom compliance officer. The essential elements of the training are five-fold. First employees must be shown the ways in which the Standard is generally carried out, such as labeling methods, warning signs, and use of Safety Data Sheets (SDSs). They must all be made aware of the health and physical hazards linked to hazardous chemicals and how they are indicated on the above. Employees must be educated in the use of appropriate personal protective equipment. The trainer must also acquaint the employee with site-specific details such as where SDSs are located, emergency procedures, protection of certain equipment, and engineering and work practice controls. Lastly, the training should include a portion where the employee observes things like the smells and appearances of specific hazardous reagents.

Chemical hygiene plan

A written chemical hygiene plan, as required by the OSHA Occupational Exposure to Hazardous Chemicals in Laboratories Standard, should cover a variety of topics. The plan should list procedures for procurement, allocation, and storage of chemicals. It should address environmental monitoring if required or in the case of problems. It should also specify housekeeping procedures such as frequency of monitoring of safety equipment (e.g., eye-face wash stations), maintenance of egress to emergency equipment, and general procedures for cleanliness. The plan should address the use of personal protective equipment and emergency equipment. PPE for chemical use is not necessarily the same as for infection control, and additional items like eye-face washes, fire extinguishers, and ventilation fume hoods are needed. The plan should address how spills and accidents are to be dealt with and evaluated thereafter. There should be a medical program in place that deals with medical surveillance, exposure outcomes, and provision of first aid. The plan should address maintenance of accident, chemical and medical records; pertinent signage (like emergency phone numbers) and labeling, training of employees, and waste disposal methods.

OSHA Occupational Exposure to Hazardous Chemicals in Laboratories Standard

The OSHA Occupational Exposure to Hazardous Chemicals in Laboratories Standard is designed to safeguard employees using hazards in a laboratory setting. It is really applicable in the dental setting to dental offices as well as dental laboratories because there are many opportunities for exposure to a hazardous chemical, defined as any chemical scientifically proven to cause acute or chronic health issues. The Standard calls for designation of a chemical hygiene officer to oversee compliance, including responsibilities such as familiarity with exposure limits, ensuring that employees use chemicals in an appropriate manner, and monitoring all facets of chemical use. It also calls for development of a written site-specific chemical hygiene plan that covers ways to protect employees against hazardous chemicals and applies the principles of prudent practices for safety and use of chemicals.

Emergency action plan

A number of OSHA standards, such as the Fire Safety Standard and the Hazard Communication Standard, require development of a written emergency action plan (EAP). Minimally the EAP should address the practices for informing authorities about a fire or other emergency, evacuation procedures and escape routes, methods of accounting for all employees after evacuation such as a designated meeting place, responsibilities of employees who might be able to perform rescue procedures such as resuscitation, and names or job classifications for contacts knowledgeable about the plan. An EAP might also include procedures for employees who stay longer than others to shut off equipment or utilities if necessary. The EAP should be gone over with each new employee. It should be available for ongoing perusal. Just as with a fire prevention plan, the EAP may be communicated verbally if there are fewer than 10 employees but a written plan is suggested as required for larger offices.

OSHA Fire Safety Standard

The OSHA Fire Safety Standard mandates that a fire safety and prevention plan be developed for the office. New employees must be informed of the components of the fire safety plan. In offices with less than 10 employees this information can be transmitted verbally, but it is suggested that a written plan be developed as is required for larger offices. The written fire safety plan should minimally include the following: an inventory of major fire hazards in the workplace; information about how possible ignition sources are used, stored and disposed of; fire protection equipment available in the office; ways that flammables and combustibles are kept to a minimum; safeguards in place on instruments that produce heat; names or job classifications of individuals responsible upkeep of equipment and control of fuel source hazards; housekeeping duties related to potential fire hazards; and components of employee training. An emergency notification and evacuation plan in case of fire should be outlined, which could also be part of an emergency action plan (discussed elsewhere). Two or more separated fire exit routes should be identified and other measures such as sprinkler systems are suggested.

Evacuation policies and procedures

As part of an emergency action plan (EAP), there are essential elements that should be included in the actual evacuation policies and procedures. The EAP should clearly single out situations that warrant evacuation (and its scope), such as fire, certain natural disasters, or chemical spills. It should identify the emergency plan coordinator and further chain of command in evacuation or shutdown situations. It should spell out how different types of emergencies should be handled. It may designate someone to shut down critical operations. It should include a map posted prominently that delineates evacuation routes and exits. It is helpful, particularly in larger workplaces, to appoint a number of employees to assist at various points during evacuations or to help visitors, people with disabilities, or those who are non-English speaking. It is also important to identify in the plan at least one assembly place after evacuation to do a head count of employees.

Issues addressed in emergency action plan

It is essential to make sure that an emergency action plan (EAP) address all potential natural or man-made emergencies, including things such as fires, natural disasters, toxic materials release, radiological and biological accidents, and interpersonal disruptions. It should also identify all potential chemical hazards and other situations that could cause emergencies. The EAP should address how emergencies might impact office operations and measures to deal with such. It should talk about the procedures for rescue operations that might be needed, such as the local fire department, and provision of necessary medical care. To the latter point, if there are not extremely close medical facilities for treatment, then personnel should receive formal first aid training. The plan should include contact information for key employees, local emergency responders, and personnel with responsibilities related to emergency action, as well as contact and medical information for all employees.

Procedures in emergency action plan

An emergency action plan (EAP) should detail procedures for alerting employees in the event of an emergency. Appropriate types of alert systems include distinctive alarm systems, announcement over a public address system, and use of floor wardens to notify and direct employees. Usually fires and other emergencies are reported to authorities by dialing "911". There may be internal methods of reporting in addition or in lieu of calling "911," such as coded intercom systems, manual pull stations, or certain alarms. In terms of employee training regarding the EAP, training should be given to new employees and everyone when the plan is initially developed, when it is altered, and annually for retraining. The training should address the following: individual responsibilities; potential hazards and appropriate actions; procedures for alerting, emergency response, evacuation, and accountability; the location of emergency equipment; and shutdown procedures if appropriate. Provisions for periodic emergency drills are also suggested.

CDC recommendations for infection control

The Centers for Disease Control (CDC) issued recommendations for infection control in the dental workplace in 2003. They are similar in many respects to the OSHA Bloodborne Pathogens Standard with the following exceptions. Many of the CDC's recommendations had to do with sterilization and disinfection of patient care items and environmental infection control. For example, the CDC suggests a central instrument processing area with areas for preparation, cleaning and decontamination, sterilization, and storage. The CDC also goes into detail about sterilization and its monitoring. The CDC recommendations cover disinfection of clinical contact surfaces with EPA-registered disinfectants, use of EPA standards for dental unit water and flushing of lines, restrictions against use of water when there are boil-water notices, and adherence to manufacturer's recommendations for decontamination of devices attached to air or water lines. The CDC suggests testing of dental office personnel for anti-HBsAg a month or two after HBV vaccination to determine effectiveness; the CDC expounds further on hand hygiene, and suggests screening for latex allergy.

<u>Unique situations</u>

In addition to some general recommendations discussed on another card, the CDC recommendations also include sections on dental radiology, administration of parenteral medications, oral surgical procedures, disposal of extracted teeth, and practices in the dental laboratory. Dental radiology infection control is covered on the Radiation Health and Safety exam. The CDC recommends use of aseptic technique and, if possible, single-dose vials when administering parenteral medications and utilization of single-use disposable devices. For oral surgical procedures, the CDC recommends hand antisepsis, use of sterile surgical gloves, and use of sterile fluids for cooling or irrigation. The CDC suggests that extracted teeth be considered medical waste, taking note of whether or not they contain amalgam. Personnel working in the dental laboratory should wear PPE and treat objects received as contaminated until appropriate measures have been taken to decontaminate these objects. CDC recommendations also talk about tuberculosis, discussed elsewhere.

CDC recommendations for microorganisms in water

The Centers for Disease Control and Prevention (CDC) currently recommends that the dental treatment output water supply in a dental office meet EPA standards for drinking water, which is less than 500 CFU/mL of heterotrophic waterborne bacteria. The dental office should refer to the dental unit manufacturer's instructions as to suitable ways to maintain and monitor this recommended quality of dental water. The office should use and follow directions related to recommended water treatment products. Personnel should discharge water and air for at least 20 to 30 seconds after each patient from any piece of equipment attached to the dental water line that has been in contact with the patient's mouth. The CDC also recommends that the dental unit manufacturer be consulted regarding regular maintenance of antiretraction devices. The desired levels of bacteria in dental water expressed above (<500 CFU/mL) are less strict than those advocated by the American Dental Association, which encourages water delivered to patients for nonsurgical procedures to be $\leq$ 200 CFU/ml. The CDC also counsels that dental unit water not be used for oral surgical procedures.

CDC Guidelines for Infection Control in Dental Health-Care Settings-2003

The Centers for Disease Control and Prevention Guidelines for Infection Control in Dental Health-Care Settings-2003 are recommendations for infection control in dental settings. These recommendations are ranked into categories IA, IB, IC, II and unresolved issues based on existing scientific data, theoretical rationale, and/or applicability. Those guidelines ranked Category IC are the most important because they are mandated by law or CDC standard to be implemented. Categories IA and IB items are strongly recommended, and Category II items are suggested. The Guidelines cover personnel health elements of an infection control program, prevention of transmission of bloodborne pathogens, hand hygiene, use of personal protective equipment, contact dermatitis and latex hypersensitivity, sterilization and disinfection of patient-care items, environmental infection control, dental unit waterlines and water quality, and a number of special considerations.

Agencies that have established or enforced guidelines for infection control

The main enforcement agency is OSHA (the Occupational Safety and Health Administration) which also has developed a number of standards to be followed, most notably for the dental office the OSHA Bloodborne Pathogens Standard and the OSHA Hazard Communication Standard. Recommendations are made by the Centers for Disease Control and Prevention (CDC), the Organization for Safety and Asepsis Procedures (OSAP), and the American Dental Association (ADA). The Food and Drug Administration (FDA) regulates manufacturing and labeling of medical devices (for example sterilizers and personal protective equipment) and solutions. The Environmental Protection Agency (EPA) approves things such as disinfecting and sterilizing solutions and also regulates hazardous waste removal.

DANB Practice Test

1. Which of the following microorganisms cannot be treated effectively with antibiotics?
    a. Streptococcus
    b. Staphylococcus aureus
    c. E. coli
    d. Epstein-Barr

2. A patient calls the morning of an appointment complaining of a fever, muscle aches, runny nose, cough, and headache. What is the appropriate action?
    a. Tell the patient he needs to come for the appointment or he will be charged for a no-show
    b. Tell the patient he may have the flu and should reschedule the appointment after the fever subsides without the use of medication
    c. Reschedule for the following day
    d. Tell the patient the decision is his to make about whether he feels up to coming in for dental work

3. Which of the following is not a likely mode of transmission for herpes simplex virus type 1?
    a. Blood
    b. Direct contact with lesion
    c. Saliva
    d. Aerosol spray from the dental handpiece

4. Which of the following is not correct regarding hepatitis B?
    a. Hepatitis B can cause serious illness involving the liver including cirrhosis, liver cancer, or liver failure
    b. Only individuals who are symptomatic can transmit the virus
    c. More than one-third of all hepatitis cases are due to hepatitis B
    d. Hepatitis B is transmitted through blood and saliva

5. What vaccination protects against lockjaw?
    a. MMR
    b. H1N1
    c. Varicella
    d. Td

6. In order for an infection to occur, 4 conditions must be present. Which of the following does not accurately describe one of these conditions?
    a. Virulence
    b. Number of microorganisms
    c. Portal of entry
    d. Any available host

7. How is tuberculosis transmitted?
    a. Airborne transmission
    b. Fecal-oral transmission
    c. Vehicular transmission
    d. Indirect transmission

8. What is the single most effective means of preventing the transmission of disease in the dental office?
    a. Use of gloves
    b. Use of mask
    c. Proper hand hygiene
    d. The use of antiseptic handwash

9. What is the recommended duration with the use of antiseptic handwash during hand hygiene?
    a. 5 seconds
    b. 15 seconds
    c. 2 minutes
    d. 5 minutes

10. Frequent handwashing can cause dryness of the hands or dermatitis. What is the best way to treat this during the work day?
    a. Avoid the use of any lotions during the work day
    b. Use of cocoa butter–based lotion
    c. Use of water-based lotion
    d. Use of petroleum-based lotion

11. A patient has a latex allergy. What should the dental assistant do for hand protection?
    a. Wear a pair of gloves made out of nitrile or polyvinyl chloride materials
    b. Put the latex gloves on and wash the gloves with soap and water before treating the patient
    c. Wash hands thoroughly with soap and water and provide treatment without the use of gloves
    d. Wear the latex gloves and monitor the patient for signs of adverse effects

12. What type of personal protective equipment (PPE) should be worn while assisting with a procedure that requires the use of a high-speed handpiece?
    a. Surgical scrubs, surgical hat, gloves, shoe covers, mask, and eye shield
    b. Surgical scrubs, gloves, and face shield
    c. Short sleeved gown, gloves, surgical mask, and eye shield
    d. Long sleeved gown, gloves, surgical mask, or face shield

13. Which of the following would be an inappropriate action regarding the use of PPE that requires laundering?
    a. Placing contaminated items that need laundering in a biohazardous waste container
    b. Taking contaminated surgical gown home for laundering following Universal Precautions
    c. Changing a gown throughout the day whenever it becomes visibly soiled
    d. Carefully removing the gown by pulling it off but keeping the gown inside out so it does not touch the clothing underneath

14. What is the name of the item used to prevent the patient from swallowing or aspirating dental debris during a procedure?
    a. Dental dam
    b. Cotton roll
    c. Dental clamp
    d. Dental arch

15. What is the basic concept that Universal or Standard Precautions is based on?
    a. Standard precautions only apply to those individuals who have a history of infectious disease
    b. Standard precautions only apply to those individuals who have a history of high-risk behavior such as drug abuse or sexual orientation
    c. Standard precautions apply to all patients and all bodily fluids should be treated as if infectious
    d. Standard precautions only apply to blood and saliva based on the patient's history

16. A dental assistant returns from the bathroom without washing hands and immediately puts on gloves. What type of disease transmission is possible?
    a. Patient to patient
    b. Patient to dental team
    c. Community to dental office
    d. Dental team to patient

17. What is the appropriate action to take when disposing of used needles in the dental office?
    a. Recap the needles using 2 hands, then dispose of in a biohazardous waste bag
    b. Handle the needles using gloves and dispose of in puncture-proof container
    c. Cut the needles into tiny pieces and dispose of in puncture-proof container
    d. Use gloves to handle the needles, put into a resealable plastic bag and dispose of in biohazardous trash

18. Which of the following would be considered an appropriate action for following aseptic technique?
    a. Removal of all jewelry
    b. Long artificial fingernails
    c. Use of steel wool to clean instruments
    d. Use of vinyl gloves during dental procedure

19. When disposing of regulated waste, what set of regulations must be followed?
    a. Local
    b. State
    c. Federal
    d. Whatever set of regulations is the most stringent

20. What type of system is used for storing clean and sterile instruments for use in specific dental procedures such as a restoration?
    a. Tub and tray system
    b. Color-coded system
    c. Preset tray system
    d. Accessory system

21. What is the term used for determining if sterilized instruments are still sterile before reuse?
    a. Event-related packaging
    b. Terminal sterilization
    c. Chemical indicator system
    d. Biological monitoring system

22. After used instruments are transferred to the instrument processing area and sorted, what is the next step in the sterilization process?
    a. Decontamination
    b. Sterilization
    c. Disinfecting
    d. Cleaning

23. The use of an autoclave for sterilization involves the use of:
    a. Dry heat
    b. Chemical vapor
    c. Steam
    d. Steam under pressure

24. Which of the following is not a chemical used in the unsaturated chemical vapor sterilization process?
    a. Acetone
    b. Ketone
    c. Glutaraldehyde
    d. Formaldehyde

25. What temperature is required for dry heat sterilization?
    a. 350°-400°F
    b. 320°-375°F
    c. 375°-450°F
    d. 400°-500°F

26. What type of sterilization monitoring is used to determine if sterilization has actually occurred?
    a. Physical monitoring
    b. Chemical monitoring
    c. Biological monitoring
    d. Physical and chemical monitoring

27. Chemical or liquid sterilization would be most appropriate for:
    a. Rubber dam equipment
    b. Clamps
    c. Condensers
    d. Stainless steel hand instruments

28. Which of the following statements is LEAST accurate regarding dental unit water lines (DUWL)?
    a. The primary source for any microorganisms present in the DUWL originates from the public water supply
    b. Water from DUWL can be used for all dental procedures
    c. Anti-retraction devices can be installed in DUWL to help prevent saliva from entering the waterline during patient care
    d. The tubing that connects the DUWL to the handpieces can become colonized with many different types of bacteria or other microorganisms

29. Clinical contact surfaces that have been contaminated by blood should be disinfected using:
   a. Liquid chemical sterilant
   b. High-level EPA registered disinfectant
   c. Intermediate-level EPA registered disinfectant
   d. Low-level EPA registered disinfectant

30. Which of the following is considered an intermediate-level disinfectant that can be used in the dental office setting?
   a. 6% hydrogen peroxide
   b. 2% alkaline glutaraldehyde
   c. Iodophors such as IodoFive
   d. Sodium hypochlorite

31. What would be an appropriate alternative for a high-level disinfectant with low odor?
   a. Isopropyl alcohol
   b. Chlorine Dioxide
   c. Glutaraldehyde
   d. Ortho-phthalaldehyde

32. Which of the following statements about isopropyl alcohol is true?
   a. Isopropyl alcohol can be used effectively as a topical skin antiseptic.
   b. Isopropyl alcohol can effectively remove blood and saliva and any microorganisms associated with these.
   c. Isopropyl alcohol has a low evaporation rate making it an effective disinfectant
   d. Isopropyl alcohol is recommended by the American Dental Association for the disinfection of environmental surfaces.

33. A low-level EPA registered disinfectant is not effective against which of the following?
   a. HIV
   b. HBV
   c. Influenza
   d. Aspergillus

34. Which of the following would NOT be considered an advantage to using surface barriers in the dental office?
   a. Efficient use of time
   b. Environmentally friendly
   c. Protection of hard to clean surfaces
   d. Provides a positive image of cleanliness to the patient

35. An advantage to using single-use disposable items in the dental office would be:
   a. More efficient for difficult to clean items
   b. Lower cost
   c. Ability to reuse the item after sterilization if desired
   d. Environmentally friendly

36. How often does the exposure control plan need to be updated?
    a. Biannually
    b. Annually
    c. Every 3 years
    d. Every 5 years

37. The term engineering controls refers to all of the following except:
    a. Sharps disposal container
    b. Self-sheaving needles
    c. Needleless systems
    d. All types of syringes

38. Which of the following would NOT be considered a work practice control?
    a. Removing the bur before taking apart the dental handpiece
    b. Avoiding the use of fingers in tissue retraction
    c. Recapping a needle using a two-handed technique
    d. Using the sharps container for disposing of used scalers

39. The OSHA Hazard Communication Standard requires all of the following EXCEPT:
    a. Provide employees with efficient access to safety data sheets for all chemicals used on site
    b. Proper training of employees regarding the use of chemicals in the workplace
    c. Provides recommendations for what chemicals to be used in certain situations
    d. Preparation of a written plan for dealing with exposure to hazardous chemicals

40. What type of documentation is required by the Occupational Safety and Health Act of 1970 for a work place injury that requires medical treatment beyond basic first aid?
    a. Report regarding the injury mailed to the employee's primary care physician
    b. Documentation by employer on a log and incident report of work-related injuries and illnesses
    c. The employer should request documentation from the emergency department or the patient's primary care physician on treatment provided for the workplace injury
    d. Ask the employee to fill out an incident report

41. What is the appropriate first-aid treatment for a chemical burn?
    a. Remove any remaining chemical and rinse the area under cool running water for 15-20 minutes
    b. Immediately put ice on the chemical injury
    c. Place Vaseline or other ointment over the chemical injury
    d. Put the area in ice cold water then cover the area with antibacterial ointment

42. What is the first step in treating a needle stick injury to a finger?
    a. Apply antibacterial ointment
    b. Apply surgical disinfectant soap
    c. Use soap and water to wash affected area as soon as possible following injury
    d. Wash with soap and water, then apply an antiseptic ointment

43. A needlestick injury has resulted in exposure to hepatitis C. Which of the following is not a recommendation for the first 6 months?
    a. Restriction from sexual activity
    b. Leave of absence from work
    c. Defer plans for starting a family
    d. Blood donation

44. What are the symptoms of nitrous oxide exposure?
    a. Difficulty breathing, headache, drowsiness
    b. Skin rash and itching
    c. Enlarged liver, abdominal pain, nausea
    d. No obvious symptoms are present

45. A patient has neglected to inform you of the development of a latex allergy. The patient begins to develop an anaphylactic reaction during dental treatment. What should be done?
    a. Remove the source of latex and allow time for the patient to recover
    b. The patient needs an injection of epinephrine; call for EMS.
    c. Call the patient's emergency contact for assistance
    d. Give the patient oxygen and call the primary care physician

46. All of the following are appropriate steps to take for protection from lasers during dental care EXCEPT for:
    a. Employee training
    b. Standard eye protection
    c. Use of matte-finish instruments
    d. Protection of outlying tissues that will not receive laser therapy with wet gauze packs

47. Which of the following would be the LEAST acceptable quality of an exit route in a dental office?
    a. The exit route should be free from stored equipment at all times
    b. The exit route should be planned so no combustible or explosive materials are stored along the way
    c. The exit route should be free of doors that are able to be locked while trying to reach an exit
    d. The quickest route out of the office

48. How long is a dental employer required to keep the records of employees?
    a. The length of employment
    b. The length of employment plus 10 years
    c. The length of employment plus 20 years
    d. The length of employment plus 30 years

49. What is the name of the law that prohibits discrimination against patients who are HIV positive?
    a. Americans with Disability Act
    b. HIV Protection Act
    c. Equal Rights Amendment
    d. HIPAA

50. Which of the following would NOT be an appropriate action for cleaning up a mercury spill?
    a. Using a piece of tape to pick up the tiny mercury droplets
    b. Using a vacuum to pick up the mercury droplets
    c. Use sulfur dust to make a film on top of the droplets until they can be adequately cleaned
    d. Use an aspirator to pick up large droplets

Answer Key and Explanations

1. D: *Streptococcus*, *Staphylococcus aureus*, and *E. coli* are all types of bacterial infections. Bacteria are tiny microorganisms that cannot be seen visually unless viewed using a microscope. Bacteria can cause different types of diseases. For example, *Streptococcus* can cause strep throat and *E. coli* can cause gastrointestinal illness due to food poisoning. Bacterial infections can be treated with different types of antibiotics depending on the type of bacteria. Epstein-Barr is a type of virus that can cause mononucleosis. Viruses cannot be treated with antibiotics. Some antiviral medications are available to treat viruses; however, most will only lessen the symptoms. Viruses typically need to run the course before symptoms are resolved.

2. B: The patient's complaint sounds like a viral illness, such as influenza. Symptoms of the seasonal flu include coughing, runny nose, muscle aches and pains, extreme fatigue, headache, and fever. The patient would be considered contagious until the fever subsides for 24 hours without the use of medication such as acetaminophen or ibuprofen. Influenza is highly contagious. The dental appointment should be rescheduled for another time after the flu has resolved. A seasonal flu vaccine is available and health care workers including dental assistants should consider getting this vaccine. The flu can be transmitted from one person to another a day before symptoms are apparent and up to a week after the flu is diagnosed. A flu vaccine protects the health care worker from getting the flu from a patient and helps to prevent transfer of the virus to patients.

3. A: Herpes is a highly contagious virus. Herpes simplex virus type 1 causes cold sores on the lips. This virus can lie dormant for a period of time. This is called a latent infection. Factors such as stress, illness, dental work, and sunlight can cause an outbreak. Transmission can occur through direct contact with lesions, infected saliva, and aerosol spray or splash back from the dental handpiece. Patients with active herpes simplex type 1 may need to reschedule dental work during an outbreak. Other types of herpes include herpes simplex virus type 2, which is genital herpes, and herpes zoster virus, which is shingles or chickenpox. All are highly contagious.

4. B: Hepatitis B virus (HBV) is an inflammation of the liver caused by a virus. HBV is spread through direct contact with blood, saliva, or other bodily fluids from a person infected with HBV. It can also be passed to an infant during childbirth. Initial infection with HBV may not cause any symptoms or may cause a prolonged illness for a few weeks before diagnosis is made. Symptoms of HBV include loss of appetite, low-grade fever, muscle pain, nausea, and vomiting. Some individuals will develop jaundice or yellowing of the skin. Even if symptoms are not present, the disease can progress and cause liver damage. Health care workers including dental assistants are at risk for contracting HBV and should give serious consideration to receiving the vaccination because of exposure to blood and saliva. The vaccination consists of 3 shots over a period of 5 months. Once the vaccination is completed, the blood can be tested to ensure antibodies are present for immunity to HBV.

5. D: Tetanus is a type of bacterial spore that is found in dirt, dust, or human waste. It is very dangerous and can be fatal is not treated. Tetanus can cause lockjaw. The symptoms of lockjaw include muscle stiffness that initially involve the jaw and neck but then progress to other parts of the body. It is very important for all health care workers to remain current on vaccinations. Td vaccination is for tetanus and diphtheria prevention in adults. Children receive this vaccination as part of the DTaP vaccination. If an adult has not received primary vaccination, this must be done by administering 3 shots on a predetermined schedule over a 6-month period. A tetanus booster must be given every 10 years.

6. D: In order for infections to occur, four conditions must be present. Virulence is the degree of strength a microorganism possesses to cause disease. Microorganisms with lower virulence will be less likely to cause an infection. The number of microorganisms is also important. Infection will not occur if there are an insufficient number of microorganisms present to invade to invade the body's defenses or immunity. There must be a portal of entry. This refers to the way the microorganism enters the body, such as a cut or inhalation. There must also be a susceptible host. The host has a weakened immune system for some reason, such as stress, presence of disease, or fatigue. Individuals who are healthy and well rested are less likely to incur an infection.

7. A: Tuberculosis (TB) is a bacterial disease that usually affects the lungs. TB is spread via airborne transmission. When an individual with TB sneezes, coughs, or even talks, droplets enter the air. These droplets can then come in contact with the respiratory tract, eyes, mouth, or nose. Small droplets can stay in the air for prolonged periods and remain capable of causing TB. Patients with active TB should be isolated and it is inappropriate for them to receive dental care in the regular office setting. Any dental office worker including dental assistants should receive a two-step baseline tuberculin skin test when starting employment. Further TB testing of employees is dependent on the level of risk determined by the number of active TB cases seen in the office every year. Low risk would be less than 3 patients with active TB. Medium risk would be 3 or more patients with active TB.

8. C: Proper hand hygiene is the most effective way to prevent the transmission of disease in the dental office. Many studies have proven this point. Noncompliance with hand hygiene increases the infection rate, spreads multi-drug-resistant organisms, and can cause outbreaks of illnesses. Proper hand hygiene should be practiced before and after treating every patient, including washing hands before and after the use of gloves. Hand hygiene is required any time a surface could be contaminated with any bodily fluid, such as blood, saliva, or respiratory secretions. Proper hand hygiene is required when leaving the dental operatory (the room where dental procedures are performed). Proper hand hygiene is required whenever hands are visibly soiled.

9. B: There are different methods for achieving good hand hygiene. The purpose of using an antiseptic hand wash is to remove or destroy microorganisms that may be present on the hands. It will also reduce the amount of resident flora, which is the species of microorganisms that are always present on the body but are less likely to cause infections. Types of antiseptic hand wash include the use of antimicrobial soap such as chlorhexidine or iodine. When using water and antimicrobial soap, the entire surface of the hands and fingers should be gently scrubbed for at least 15 seconds. Routine hand washing can be accomplished using water and regular soap. This can be followed up with the use of an antiseptic hand rub.

10. C: Continued hand washing throughout the work day is likely to cause dryness of the skin or dermatitis. Because one of the points of entry for infection is cuts on the skin, it is extremely important to take care of the skin. Petroleum-based lotions can interfere with the protection of latex gloves by weakening the structure and increasing permeability. Lotions containing petroleum or other emollients, such as cocoa butter, should be used outside of the dental office. If lotion is required during the work day, it is best to choose a water-based lotion that will not interact with gloves.

11. A: There are many different types of gloves available. Not using gloves during treatment is not an option for both the operator and the patient's protection. Washing latex gloves is never a good idea because this can cause tiny punctures in the gloves. These tiny holes allow liquid to enter into the gloves in a process called wicking. For anyone with a latex allergy, the use of nitrile, polyvinyl

chloride, or polyethylene gloves should be substituted. Many dental offices are beginning to transition to latex-free gloves because of the increase in latex allergies for patients and employees.

12. D: Personal protective equipment (PPE) needs to be provided according to the OSHA Bloodborne Pathogens (BBP) Standard. PPE includes protective clothing such as gowns or lab coats, surgical masks, appropriate gloves, face shield, and protective eye wear. Dental assistants should wear the appropriate PPE depending upon the procedure being performed. This will help to protect against contact with blood, saliva, aerosol, spray, or any other material. PPE must also be worn when handling items that may be contaminated, such as dentures, extracted teeth, or contaminated equipment. When using a high speed handpiece, it is important to wear the appropriate clothing. This would consist of a long-sleeved gown, gloves, surgical mask, and eye wear or a protective face shield. The face shield would protect against spray or splatter entering the body through parts of the face.

13. B: The OSHA BBP regulations prohibit any contaminated laundry form being removed from the dental office for cleaning in the home setting. Contaminated laundry may include surgical nondisposable gowns, cloths or towels, or washcloths. Contaminated laundry needs to be bagged in a leak-proof bag that has the biohazard label affixed to the bag. Protective clothing should never be worn outside of the dental office because of the risk of cross contamination. Protective clothing should be changed whenever an item becomes visibly soiled with blood, saliva, etc. Protective clothing should not be changed around others who are eating or working. Gowns should be removed and turned inside out while removing so the clothing underneath does not get contaminated.

14. A: A dental dam is an important item used in infection control for patients. It helps to protect the patient from swallowing or aspirating pieces of tooth or other types of infectious dental debris. It also helps to prevent the exposed tooth from contamination while a procedure is occurring. The dental dam also functions in the retraction of the lips, tongue, and gums from the area of operation. The dental dam consists of either latex or silicone flexible material that varies in size, color, and thickness, a dam frame, napkin, lubricant, and dam punch. The dam punch provides a way to expose the tooth or teeth involved in the procedure. A dental clamp is also used in this process to hold the dam in place.

15. C: The Centers for Disease Control and Prevention (CDC) developed Standard Precautions to help prevent the spread of disease. Standard Precautions and Universal Precautions are used interchangeably. The basic concept for Universal or Standard Precautions is that all blood and bodily fluids should be treated as infectious. It is not possible to determine which patients may have an infectious illness even with the patient's history available for review. Some patients do not tell the truth and some patients might not know about a condition. Universal or Standard Precautions should apply to all patients. Bodily fluids that may spread disease include blood, secretions, saliva, skin, mucous membranes, and products of excretion. Standard Precautions consist of handwashing, the use of personal protective equipment, treatment of patient care equipment and environmental surfaces, and prevention of injury.

16. D: Failure to wash hands after using the bathroom may result in transmission of microorganisms via fecal-oral route. Transfer may then occur from the dental team (the dental assistant that did not wash hands) to the patient. Since many pathogens are present in human excrement, it is possible to transmit a number of diseases this way, including hepatitis A, rotavirus, and *Clostridium difficile*. The lack of handwashing could potentially contaminate a number of surfaces along the way back to the operatory, such as door handles, light switches, pens, and computer keyboards. Another way for disease transmission to occur would be patient to dental

team (most common), patient to patient, dental office to community, and community to dental office to patient.

17. B: Sharps include needles, wires, scalpel blades, and any other potentially sharp object. Sharps that are contaminated with any bodily fluid must be considered hazardous waste and treated in a specialized manner. Recapping of needles is not recommended. If this must occur, it should be done using one hand in a specialized technique that should be practiced before it is performed. Needles should never be broken, bent, or cut. Sharps should only be disposed of in a puncture-proof container. These containers should be labeled with the biohazard symbol, should be located close to the work station in the dental operatory, and should be constructed to prevent anyone from entering into the container once the sharp has been inserted. Each state has regulations dictating the frequency of pickup of the sharps containers.

18. A: Aseptic technique refers to a set of procedures used to minimize contamination by pathogens. There are controlled steps to achieve asepsis. Handwashing is always the very first step in aseptic technique. The use of personal protective equipment is also included. Equipment and supplies must also be treated in an aseptic manner to prevent contamination. The use of environmental barriers is recommended, such as clear wrap over frequently used items (for example, computer keyboards). All items within the sterile field in the operatory must be sterile. Any contaminated item must be removed immediately to prevent cross-contamination. Safe disposal of all medical waste is essential. When preparing for aseptic technique, dental assistants should remove all jewelry, and fingernails should be short and well-manicured. Long or artificial nails are not recommended because of the possibility of bacteria getting under the nails. Only latex gloves or other approved surgical gloves should be used. Steel wool is not used on the cleaning of any equipment.

19. D: The Environmental Protection Agency (EPA) is responsible for enforcing the regulations for regulated waste. Regulated waste includes sharps, such as disposable needles, broken glass contaminated with potentially infectious materials, scrap amalgam, x-ray fixer or developer solutions, and mercury-containing products. Regulated waste also encompasses blood or blood contaminated products, and pathological waste, such as human tissue. The dental office must follow whatever regulations are the most stringent among local, state, or federal authorities. The dental office is responsible for labeling the regulated waste appropriately, packaging and storing the waste, and arranging for a licensed waste disposal service to take care of the waste. The dentist is ultimately responsible for making sure regulated waste is taken care of legally.

20. C: Hand instruments and accessories for a specific dental procedure, such as a restoration, can be kept together as a set. These instruments are cleaned and sterilized at the same time. The items are then placed into a tray or cassette and sealed. This type of system is known as a preset tray or preset cassette system. The tray is then brought into the operatory when needed for a patient's procedure. Another type of system that can be used for dental instrument storage is a color-coded system. Various colors are used depending upon the type of function or procedure the instrument is used for. The tray can also be color coded for easy of identification. A tub and tray system uses a plastic tub that is covered but contains all the instruments needed for a specific procedure. Whichever system for storing instruments is used, the most important point is to follow proper infection control guidelines before and after the use of instruments.

21. A: Event-related packaging is the way in which sterilized dental instruments are packaged. Once the clean instruments are wrapped and then sterilized, the assumption is that the tools will remain sterile unless an event occurs. The event could be that the packaging is torn or open or becomes wet. The outside of the wrapping should indicate the date of sterilization. Information regarding the

exact sterilizer used could also be included if there is more than one sterilizer in the dental office. Wrapped and sterile instruments should be appropriately stored in a closed cabinet. These items should never be stored under an open cabinet or near a sink.

22. D: All instruments and equipment that are reusable should be treated in one central processing area, typically called an instrument processing area. This area should be divided into four distinct sections that separate out items to be cleaned, prepared and packaged, sterilized, and storage. These areas should have a physical barrier separating them from each other. Once the used items are in the first area, they are sorted. The next step should be cleaning. This step occurs before any disinfecting or sterilizing takes place. Cleaning involves the removal of any visible material, such as blood. This can be accomplished using a brush with surfactant, detergent, and water. After the items are cleaned, they should be thoroughly rinsed with clean water. Alternatively, items can be placed to soak in an enzymatic cleaner or a detergent/disinfectant solution if manual cleaning cannot happen immediately. This step prevents material from drying on the instruments.

23. D: An autoclave is often used for sterilization of dental instruments. The sterilization process occurs with the use of pressurized steam. Items to be sterilized must be cleaned and then wrapped before being paced in the autoclave. There are 4 cycles in the autoclaving process. The first is the heat up cycle. The water in the autoclave is heated to a high enough temperature to produce steam, which in turn produces moist heat. The second cycle is the sterilization cycle. This temperature needs to be between 250° and 273°F, depending upon the length of this step. This moist heat is strong enough to kill any microorganisms present. The third cycle is the depressurization cycle and the last cycle is the drying cycle. It is important to allow all items to cool and dry before removing from the autoclave. Serious injury can occur if items are immediately handled because of the high temperatures used in the sterilization process.

24. C: Another type of sterilization is called unsaturated chemical vapor sterilization. It is similar to autoclaving but instead uses a combination of chemicals to form a vapor that causes sterilization. The chemicals involved are alcohol, formaldehyde, ketone, and acetone. Water is also used. Employees involved in this process must wear the appropriate personal protective equipment because of the toxicity of the chemicals. The instruments to be sterilized must be both cleaned and dried before they are wrapped. The chemical vapor sterilizer is loaded according to the manufacturer's direction. The controls are set to encompass the correct pressure, time, and temperature to achieve sterility. Instruments must be cooled before removing from the sterilizer. The advantage to this process is the instruments do not rust, corrode, or alter the sharpness of the instruments. The disadvantage is that the chemical vapors that are produced with the sterilization process are toxic and proper venting is essential to prevent personal injury.

25. B: Dry heat sterilization is another type of sterilization process that is commonly used in dental offices. Air is heated to a temperature between 320° and 375°F. The exact temperature depends upon the length of the sterilization cycle. There are 2 types of dry heat sterilizers, static air and forced air. Static air works like a convection oven while the forced air sterilizer works by circulating hot air at a high rate of speed throughout the heat chamber. Items to be sterilized must be cleaned and dried before being wrapped. If the items are not dry before using dry heat sterilization, the instruments will rust. Any instrument with a hinge, such as scissors or forceps, should be in the open position. The heat chamber is loaded and the temperature and time controls are set according to manufacturer's directions. Cooling must take placed before any of the wrapped packages are handled because of the risk of serious burn injury.

26. C: There are 3 types of methods available for sterilization monitoring, physical, chemical, and biological. Biological monitoring is the only type that determines if sterilization actually occurred.

At the minimum, weekly biological testing is recommended by the American Dental Association and the Centers for Disease Control and Prevention (CDC). This type of monitoring involves the testing for spores such as *Geobacillus* or *Bacillus* species. The absence of these resistant spores would indicate all pathogens have been effectively killed. Physical monitoring involves monitoring and recording readings on the sterilizer for temperature, exposure time, and pressure. Chemical monitoring involves using a heat-sensitive chemical that changes color in response to conditions inside or outside the sterilizer. Process indicators are used outside to confirm if appropriate temperatures have been reached but do not check duration or pressure. Process integrators are used inside the instrument packages and will measure pressure, temperature, and duration. This may involve the use of strips or tubes of colored liquid. Neither physical nor chemical monitoring will guarantee sterility.

27. A: Some items used for dental care are not heat tolerant but still require sterilization. These items may include rubber dam equipment, some x-ray film holding apparatuses, and other hand instruments that may contain rubber. In this situation, a liquid chemical sterilant must be selected. A liquid sterilant or sterilizing agent is used that is 2% to 3.4% glutaraldehyde. This requires at least 10 hours of contact time in order to be considered sterile. Less than 10 hours would only be considered disinfected. Care must be taken when working with glutaraldehyde because of the toxic nature of the fumes. Personal protective equipment including utility gloves, masks, gowns, and eye wear must be worn.

28. B: The contamination of dental unit water lines (DUWL) can be an issue in dental offices. This is of particular concern because immunocompromised patients may become ill from contaminated water. The source of contamination can be from both the public water supply entering the DUWL and from the patient's mouth during dental care. Colonization can also occur in the tubing. Installation of anti-retraction devices can help reduce contamination as well as flushing the DUWL between patients. The public water supply is usually safe and must adhere to specific standards; however, when this water enters the DUWL, it mixes with other microorganisms and these can begin to multiply. DUWL can be used during most dental procedures except for surgical procedures involving the mouth. Sterile water should be used in this case. Occasionally, a boil water advisory will be issued for a public water supply and the DUWL should not be used in this situation. There are a couple different ways that DUWL can be tested and monitored for safety, including in-office test kits.

29. C: There are 3 categories for clinical contamination. Touch surfaces are surfaces that are contaminated during treatment. The surfaces would include dental unit controls, light handles, computers by the dental chair, containers holding dental materials, drawer handles, and other areas. Transfer surfaces are not touched routinely but may come in contact with contaminated instruments, such as instrument trays. Splash, splatter, and droplet surfaces are not in actual contact with contaminated items but may inadvertently become contaminated during treatment. Any area that becomes contaminated with blood should be disinfected with an intermediate-level EPA registered disinfectant. A low-level disinfectant will not disinfect appropriately and liquid chemical sterilants or high-level disinfectants should not be used for surface cleaning.

30. C: Intermediate-level disinfectants are able to inactivate *Mycobacterium tuberculosis*. Intermediate-level disinfectants do not kill bacterial spores. A high-level disinfectant is required to kill bacteria spores. Types of intermediate-level disinfectants that are approved for use in dental offices include phenolics, iodophors, and chlorine-containing compounds. Synthetic phenols compounds are approved for broad-spectrum disinfecting and can be used on a variety of surfaces including metal, glass, plastic, or rubber. Iodophors contain iodine and also have broad-spectrum activity. This product may cause discoloration of some surfaces. Sodium hypochlorite is household

bleach. It is considered an intermediate-level disinfectant; however, it is no longer approved by the EPA for use in dental offices. Other approved products that contain chlorines may be used.

31. D: A high-level disinfectant registered with the EPA is required for semi-critical dental instruments that are not heat tolerant. This would include items such as mirrors, amalgam condensers, and reusable trays. A high-level disinfectant must be capable of killing spores. Glutaraldehyde is the most commonly used high-level disinfectant; however, many people are sensitive to the fumes. The amount of time required for disinfection is up to 90 minutes. Chlorine dioxide is another high-level disinfectant; however, it must also be used with good ventilation because of its odorous fumes. Ortho-phthalaldehyde is an appropriate alternative. This product will disinfect within 12 minutes and has a low odor. The disadvantage is that this product is more expensive than other high-level disinfectants.

32. A: Isopropyl alcohol is commonly used as a topical skin antiseptic. It is added to hand sanitizer and is mistakenly used to disinfect certain types of medical equipment. Although isopropyl alcohol is considered bactericidal (capable of killing bacteria), it is not considered bacteriostatic (able to inhibit the growth of bacteria). Isopropyl alcohol and ethyl alcohol are not effective against bacterial spores or certain types of viruses. Alcohols are not effective at removing any microorganisms associated with blood or saliva. Alcohol tends to require a longer length of time in order to be effective; however, it evaporates quickly. Alcohols will also damage certain types of materials, such as rubber and plastics. Alcohols are also highly flammable.

33. D: Low-level disinfectants registered with the EPA include products such as quaternary ammonium compounds. These products are able to inactivate certain types of bacteria, fungi, and viruses. Types would include HIV, herpes simplex virus, and hepatitis B and C: It would also be effective against *Staphylococcus, Pseudomonas,* and *Salmonella* species. *Aspergillus* and *Candida,* both types of fungi, would require an intermediate-level disinfectant, as would polio, Coxsackie virus, and rhinovirus. Research has not demonstrated that floors or walls play a significant role in disease transmission; however, these surfaces need to be effectively cleaned. It is important to make fresh cleaning solution daily to prevent microorganisms from multiplying in dirty buckets.

34. B: Many surfaces in the operatory are difficult to clean. The invention of surface barrier protection has improved the ability to protect and maintain surfaces, such as knobs, handles for certain dental instruments, light switches, touch pads on equipment, and computer keyboards. These areas must continue to be cleaned and disinfected at the start and end of the workday even with the use of barriers. Barriers must be changed between patients. Advantages include a reduction in time spent cleaning and disinfecting the operatory between patients, reduction in the use of chemicals, and less damage to equipment due to moisture and chemicals. It also provides the patient with the visualization of a clean area during dental treatment. Surface barriers are not environmentally friendly because they are not able to be recycled and must be discarded in the appropriate waste container (typically unregulated unless visibly soiled with blood).

35. A: Single-use or disposable items are popular in the dental operatory for certain types of items that may be difficult to clean. This may increase efficiency in terms of time savings and sterility. Single-use items must never be reused. These items are usually made of lower grade materials, such as plastic or less costly metals, and cannot withstand the process of sterilization. Certain items are always disposable, such as cups and brushes, patient napkins, syringes used for irrigation, masks, gloves, needles used for sutures, and the sharps container. Other items are available as single use or reusable. These items may include mirrors, certain angles, burs, air water syringe tips, high-volume evacuator tips, and impression trays. Most items that are disposable can be discarded in the regular office trash unless significant blood is present.

36. B: Title 29 of the Code of Federal Regulations requires that an exposure control plan be established to protect workers who may be occupationally exposed to blood or other potentially infectious materials (OPIM). The plan details how the employer plans to minimize the risks for exposure. The plan also details who may be at risk within the workplace and what tasks or procedures may result in an exposure. The plan must be updated every year. The update should encompass any changes in procedures or tasks that may directly affect occupational exposure. The employer also needs to have documentation that safer medical devices have been researched that may reduce the risk of occupational exposure. The update must also show that input has been obtained from employees who are at risk for occupational exposure in terms of any changes that are needed to the exposure control plan.

37. D: Engineering controls in dentistry refer to the types of available items that reduce or remove the risk of exposure to a bloodborne pathogen due to sharp instruments in the workplace. Engineering controls help to address these hazards using items such as the sharps disposal container, which securely stores used needles and prevents accidental needle sticks. It also encompasses items such as needleless systems, which remove most needles from practice, or self-sheathing needles, which have a cover that slides back over the needle after use. Any medical device that is implemented to reduce the potential for exposure is considered an engineering control.

38. C: Work practice controls are practices or procedures that are developed to protect the dental health care provider from accidental injury from a sharp or other contaminated item. It defines the proper way to perform certain tasks. This would include the removal of burs before the dental handpiece is taken apart for cleaning and sterilizing, and how to handle needles, scalers, utility knives, and other sharp instruments safely. Work practice controls also prohibit the use of fingers for tissue retraction or when performing sutures. Specifications for handling dirty laundry and for cleaning contaminated surfaces are covered under work practice controls. Using a two-handed technique for recapping needles is not recommended. A one-handed "scoop" technique is the preferred work practice control

39. C: The basic premise of the OSHA Hazard Communication Standard is that employees have the right to know what type of chemicals they may be exposed to in the workplace. Employees must have access to the protective measures that are available to them and proper procedures for working with these chemicals. The first step is the identification of all chemicals in the workplace by preparing safety data sheets. There are regulations regarding the preparation of these sheets and the labeling of the chemical containers. Theses sheets will provide information from the manufacturer about the different properties of the chemical, proper disposal, first-aid treatment, etc. A Hazard Communication Program must also be implemented and employees must have easy access to this plan. Employee training is also required. The Hazard Communication Standard does not tell employers what chemicals should be used for different situations.

40. B: OSHA requires that employees work in a safe and healthy environment. Accidents and injuries do happen on the job and OSHA requires employers to provide first-aid medical care if indicated and properly document the injury. OSHA Form 300 and 301 or forms similar to these must be completed within 7 days of an employee injury. Form 300 is a log that lists specific details about individual injuries, including the employee's name, date of injury, place of injury, description of injury or illness, number of days the employee was affected by the injury or illness, and end result (if any) of the injury or illness. Form 301 is an injury and illness incident report that documents information about the employee affected, as well as medical treatment received and circumstances and details surrounding the injury.

41. A: If a chemical burn occurs in the workplace, any remaining dry chemical should be gently removed from the skin. The affected area should then be placed under cool running water for 10-20 minutes. Any jewelry or clothing that was in contact with the chemical should be removed. After the area has been rinsed, the burned area should be gently dried and covered with a dry sterile dressing. The area should be rewashed as needed if additional burning occurs. Ice, ointments, or other treatments are not recommended. An over-the-counter pain reliever may be given and a tetanus shot may be required. Chemical burns that penetrate through the first later of skin should receive immediate medical care. Chemical burns to the eye, hands, face, groin area, or major joint should also receive immediate medical care.

42. C: The first step in treating a needlestick injury is to thoroughly wash the affected area with soap and water. If the injury was to the eye, the eye should be flushed with water or saline. Antiseptic products or disinfectants should not be applied. After the injury has been cleaned, it must be reported and documented. The report must detail the date and time of exposure and how the incident occurred. Details regarding the amount of fluid exposed and severity should also be documented. The third step is to evaluate the exposure for risk of contraction of HBV, HCV, or HIV. A needlestick injury would involve blood. The fourth step is to evaluate the exposure source. If the source patient is known, request permission to screen for bloodborne pathogens. The final step is disease-specific management. For example, if the source patient tests positive for any bloodborne pathogen, then the affected employee should be treated accordingly.

43. D: The last step in the Post-Exposure Prophylaxis is follow-up. If exposed to hepatitis C, follow-up testing for hepatitis C virus and liver function tests will need to be done at approximately 4-6 months. A test for HCV RNA can be done sooner at 4-6 weeks; however, this test can sometimes yield a false-positive. During the follow-up period, the affected employee should be asked not to donate blood, plasma, any organs, or semen. Changes in daily activities do not need to be made, such as restriction from sexual activity. Plans for breastfeeding or pregnancy can continue as desired. Mental health counseling can be offered for those that may be having a hard time dealing with the situation.

44. A: Exposure to nitrous oxide is a possibility in the dental operatory. Nitrous oxide is a colorless gas that has a sweet odor. Symptoms of exposure may include headache, difficulty breathing, and drowsiness. It can also cause frostbite in the liquid form. If the exposure is due to inhalation, the affected person should be moved to fresh air and given oxygen as needed. Medical care may be required if breathing remains difficult. Exposure to eyes would require immediate flushing of the eyes with water and seeking medical care immediately. Exposure to the skin would require immediate cleansing with soap and water. Contaminated clothing should be removed immediately. Medical care should be obtained if skin irritation continues after initial treatment.

45. B: A latex allergy is a reaction to certain proteins found in natural latex. Mild allergic symptoms can include itching of the skin, redness, and a rash. If the symptoms are more severe, sneezing, wheezing, cough, runny nose, or itchy eyes may occur. The allergic reaction may progress to anaphylaxis, with difficulty breathing, reduction in blood pressure, weak pulse, and possible loss of consciousness. If an anaphylactic reaction occurs, emergency medical care should be obtained immediately. The patient will require an injection of epinephrine. If epinephrine is available, it should be administered according to instructions while waiting for EMS to arrive. It is extremely important to obtain updated allergy information from patients to help prevent this type of occurrence.

46. B: A laser beam is an extremely concentrated source of light used to cut or cauterize tissues. It is also used to vaporize or eliminate tissue. Lasers are sometimes used in dentistry for preparing a

tooth for filling, to reshape gums, and for bacterial removal prior to root canal. Lasers can also be used for teeth whitening and for biopsies. Laser therapy can have adverse effects for both the patient and the dental worker. Training must be provided in the use of laser therapy and for safety precautions. Special (not standard) eye protection must be worn that protects the eyes and signs must be posted warning that lasers are in use. Using instruments made with a matte finish instead of a shiny finish can help to prevent reflection of the laser beams. Wet gauze packs are used to shield tissues around the area being treated to protect them from laser damage. Additionally, high-volume evacuators need to be used to capture the plume or vapors as the tissue is targeted.

47. D: The quickest route out of the dental office is not always the safest. OSHA has a set of regulations governing the features of an exit route out of the dental office. Exit routes need to be carefully planned away from areas where hazardous materials are stored. There should be no potentially explosive or combustible materials in the path. Equipment should be properly stored at all times and away from the exit route. The exit route should never go through any door that has the capability to be locked and should not exit into any dead-end location. All doors should be clearly marked with "exit," "not an exit," or the function of the room, such as closet. Sprinkler systems and other safety measures should always be in good working order.

48. D: The dental office employer must keep records for each employee for the length of employment plus 30 years. The records must be confidential and kept in a locked location. The records include medical information, including accidental injuries or accidents that occurred at the worksite. The records also must contain immunization records. Employee records also contain a history of earnings, tax information, workers compensation information, and other types of information. This is an OSHA requirement. If the dental practice is sold, all employee records become the legal property of the new owner.

49. A: The Americans with Disabilities Act is a comprehensive act that covers both patients and employees. The law was written to prevent the discrimination of any handicapped person. The law prevents discrimination of a disabled person for hiring purposes. It also requires that reasonable accommodations be made to address disabilities. This means the dental office must be handicap accessible for both patients and employees who may be handicapped. Disabilities can include patients with AIDS or HIV. Adherence to standard precautions within the dental office will provide reasonable protection from infectious diseases. Other disabilities would include cancer, diabetes, heart disease, wheelchair bound, mental illness, and other types of conditions.

50. B: Mercury can be found in dental offices in amalgam. Even small amounts of mercury can be toxic. Mercury can be inhaled or absorbed through the skin. Mercury spill kits should be readily available for cleanup if needed. The spill kit contains an aspirator, a bottle to store the spilled mercury in, and specific products that will help to absorb small amounts of mercury or absorb the vapors. A product such as sulfur dust can be used to help contain the droplets if the spill occurs in a hard to reach place. Scoops, special sponges, and a special polyethylene bag for disposal are also included in the kit. Proper disposal according to regulations is required. Neither a vacuum cleaner nor a high-volume evacuator should be used in the cleanup process. The use of either of these would release toxic vapors into the air, posing a danger to anyone in the area.

How to Overcome Test Anxiety

Just the thought of taking a test is enough to make most people a little nervous. A test is an important event that can have a long-term impact on your future, so it's important to take it seriously and it's natural to feel anxious about performing well. But just because anxiety is normal, that doesn't mean that it's helpful in test taking, or that you should simply accept it as part of your life. Anxiety can have a variety of effects. These effects can be mild, like making you feel slightly nervous, or severe, like blocking your ability to focus or remember even a simple detail.

If you experience test anxiety—whether severe or mild—it's important to know how to beat it. To discover this, first you need to understand what causes test anxiety.

Causes of Test Anxiety

While we often think of anxiety as an uncontrollable emotional state, it can actually be caused by simple, practical things. One of the most common causes of test anxiety is that a person does not feel adequately prepared for their test. This feeling can be the result of many different issues such as poor study habits or lack of organization, but the most common culprit is time management. Starting to study too late, failing to organize your study time to cover all of the material, or being distracted while you study will mean that you're not well prepared for the test. This may lead to cramming the night before, which will cause you to be physically and mentally exhausted for the test. Poor time management also contributes to feelings of stress, fear, and hopelessness as you realize you are not well prepared but don't know what to do about it.

Other times, test anxiety is not related to your preparation for the test but comes from unresolved fear. This may be a past failure on a test, or poor performance on tests in general. It may come from comparing yourself to others who seem to be performing better or from the stress of living up to expectations. Anxiety may be driven by fears of the future—how failure on this test would affect your educational and career goals. These fears are often completely irrational, but they can still negatively impact your test performance.

Review Video: 3 Reasons You Have Test Anxiety
Visit mometrix.com/academy and enter code: 428468

Elements of Test Anxiety

As mentioned earlier, test anxiety is considered to be an emotional state, but it has physical and mental components as well. Sometimes you may not even realize that you are suffering from test anxiety until you notice the physical symptoms. These can include trembling hands, rapid heartbeat, sweating, nausea, and tense muscles. Extreme anxiety may lead to fainting or vomiting. Obviously, any of these symptoms can have a negative impact on testing. It is important to recognize them as soon as they begin to occur so that you can address the problem before it damages your performance.

> **Review Video: 3 Ways to Tell You Have Test Anxiety**
> Visit mometrix.com/academy and enter code: 927847

The mental components of test anxiety include trouble focusing and inability to remember learned information. During a test, your mind is on high alert, which can help you recall information and stay focused for an extended period of time. However, anxiety interferes with your mind's natural processes, causing you to blank out, even on the questions you know well. The strain of testing during anxiety makes it difficult to stay focused, especially on a test that may take several hours. Extreme anxiety can take a huge mental toll, making it difficult not only to recall test information but even to understand the test questions or pull your thoughts together.

> **Review Video: How Test Anxiety Affects Memory**
> Visit mometrix.com/academy and enter code: 609003

Effects of Test Anxiety

Test anxiety is like a disease—if left untreated, it will get progressively worse. Anxiety leads to poor performance, and this reinforces the feelings of fear and failure, which in turn lead to poor performances on subsequent tests. It can grow from a mild nervousness to a crippling condition. If allowed to progress, test anxiety can have a big impact on your schooling, and consequently on your future.

Test anxiety can spread to other parts of your life. Anxiety on tests can become anxiety in any stressful situation, and blanking on a test can turn into panicking in a job situation. But fortunately, you don't have to let anxiety rule your testing and determine your grades. There are a number of relatively simple steps you can take to move past anxiety and function normally on a test and in the rest of life.

> **Review Video: How Test Anxiety Impacts Your Grades**
> Visit mometrix.com/academy and enter code: 939819

Physical Steps for Beating Test Anxiety

While test anxiety is a serious problem, the good news is that it can be overcome. It doesn't have to control your ability to think and remember information. While it may take time, you can begin taking steps today to beat anxiety.

Just as your first hint that you may be struggling with anxiety comes from the physical symptoms, the first step to treating it is also physical. Rest is crucial for having a clear, strong mind. If you are tired, it is much easier to give in to anxiety. But if you establish good sleep habits, your body and mind will be ready to perform optimally, without the strain of exhaustion. Additionally, sleeping well helps you to retain information better, so you're more likely to recall the answers when you see the test questions.

Getting good sleep means more than going to bed on time. It's important to allow your brain time to relax. Take study breaks from time to time so it doesn't get overworked, and don't study right before bed. Take time to rest your mind before trying to rest your body, or you may find it difficult to fall asleep.

> **Review Video: The Importance of Sleep for Your Brain**
> Visit mometrix.com/academy and enter code: 319338

Along with sleep, other aspects of physical health are important in preparing for a test. Good nutrition is vital for good brain function. Sugary foods and drinks may give a burst of energy but this burst is followed by a crash, both physically and emotionally. Instead, fuel your body with protein and vitamin-rich foods.

Also, drink plenty of water. Dehydration can lead to headaches and exhaustion, especially if your brain is already under stress from the rigors of the test. Particularly if your test is a long one, drink water during the breaks. And if possible, take an energy-boosting snack to eat between sections.

> **Review Video: How Diet Can Affect your Mood**
> Visit mometrix.com/academy and enter code: 624317

Along with sleep and diet, a third important part of physical health is exercise. Maintaining a steady workout schedule is helpful, but even taking 5-minute study breaks to walk can help get your blood pumping faster and clear your head. Exercise also releases endorphins, which contribute to a positive feeling and can help combat test anxiety.

When you nurture your physical health, you are also contributing to your mental health. If your body is healthy, your mind is much more likely to be healthy as well. So take time to rest, nourish your body with healthy food and water, and get moving as much as possible. Taking these physical steps will make you stronger and more able to take the mental steps necessary to overcome test anxiety.

> **Review Video: How to Stay Healthy and Prevent Test Anxiety**
> Visit mometrix.com/academy and enter code: 877894

Mental Steps for Beating Test Anxiety

Working on the mental side of test anxiety can be more challenging, but as with the physical side, there are clear steps you can take to overcome it. As mentioned earlier, test anxiety often stems from lack of preparation, so the obvious solution is to prepare for the test. Effective studying may be the most important weapon you have for beating test anxiety, but you can and should employ several other mental tools to combat fear.

First, boost your confidence by reminding yourself of past success—tests or projects that you aced. If you're putting as much effort into preparing for this test as you did for those, there's no reason you should expect to fail here. Work hard to prepare; then trust your preparation.

Second, surround yourself with encouraging people. It can be helpful to find a study group, but be sure that the people you're around will encourage a positive attitude. If you spend time with others who are anxious or cynical, this will only contribute to your own anxiety. Look for others who are motivated to study hard from a desire to succeed, not from a fear of failure.

Third, reward yourself. A test is physically and mentally tiring, even without anxiety, and it can be helpful to have something to look forward to. Plan an activity following the test, regardless of the outcome, such as going to a movie or getting ice cream.

When you are taking the test, if you find yourself beginning to feel anxious, remind yourself that you know the material. Visualize successfully completing the test. Then take a few deep, relaxing breaths and return to it. Work through the questions carefully but with confidence, knowing that you are capable of succeeding.

Developing a healthy mental approach to test taking will also aid in other areas of life. Test anxiety affects more than just the actual test—it can be damaging to your mental health and even contribute to depression. It's important to beat test anxiety before it becomes a problem for more than testing.

> **Review Video:** **Test Anxiety and Depression**
> Visit mometrix.com/academy and enter code: 904704

Study Strategy

Being prepared for the test is necessary to combat anxiety, but what does being prepared look like? You may study for hours on end and still not feel prepared. What you need is a strategy for test prep. The next few pages outline our recommended steps to help you plan out and conquer the challenge of preparation.

Step 1: Scope Out the Test

Learn everything you can about the format (multiple choice, essay, etc.) and what will be on the test. Gather any study materials, course outlines, or sample exams that may be available. Not only will this help you to prepare, but knowing what to expect can help to alleviate test anxiety.

Step 2: Map Out the Material

Look through the textbook or study guide and make note of how many chapters or sections it has. Then divide these over the time you have. For example, if a book has 15 chapters and you have five days to study, you need to cover three chapters each day. Even better, if you have the time, leave an extra day at the end for overall review after you have gone through the material in depth.

If time is limited, you may need to prioritize the material. Look through it and make note of which sections you think you already have a good grasp on, and which need review. While you are studying, skim quickly through the familiar sections and take more time on the challenging parts. Write out your plan so you don't get lost as you go. Having a written plan also helps you feel more in control of the study, so anxiety is less likely to arise from feeling overwhelmed at the amount to cover. A sample plan may look like this:

- Day 1: Skim chapters 1–4, study chapter 5 (especially pages 31–33)
- Day 2: Study chapters 6–7, skim chapters 8–9
- Day 3: Skim chapter 10, study chapters 11–12 (especially pages 87–90)
- Day 4: Study chapters 13–15
- Day 5: Overall review (focus most on chapters 5, 6, and 12), take practice test

Step 3: Gather Your Tools

Decide what study method works best for you. Do you prefer to highlight in the book as you study and then go back over the highlighted portions? Or do you type out notes of the important information? Or is it helpful to make flashcards that you can carry with you? Assemble the pens, index cards, highlighters, post-it notes, and any other materials you may need so you won't be distracted by getting up to find things while you study.

If you're having a hard time retaining the information or organizing your notes, experiment with different methods. For example, try color-coding by subject with colored pens, highlighters, or post-it notes. If you learn better by hearing, try recording yourself reading your notes so you can listen while in the car, working out, or simply sitting at your desk. Ask a friend to quiz you from your flashcards, or try teaching someone the material to solidify it in your mind.

Step 4: Create Your Environment

It's important to avoid distractions while you study. This includes both the obvious distractions like visitors and the subtle distractions like an uncomfortable chair (or a too-comfortable couch that makes you want to fall asleep). Set up the best study environment possible: good lighting and a comfortable work area. If background music helps you focus, you may want to turn it on, but otherwise keep the room quiet. If you are using a computer to take notes, be sure you don't have any other windows open, especially applications like social media, games, or anything else that could distract you. Silence your phone and turn off notifications. Be sure to keep water close by so you stay hydrated while you study (but avoid unhealthy drinks and snacks).

Also, take into account the best time of day to study. Are you freshest first thing in the morning? Try to set aside some time then to work through the material. Is your mind clearer in the afternoon or evening? Schedule your study session then. Another method is to study at the same time of day that you will take the test, so that your brain gets used to working on the material at that time and will be ready to focus at test time.

Step 5: Study!

Once you have done all the study preparation, it's time to settle into the actual studying. Sit down, take a few moments to settle your mind so you can focus, and begin to follow your study plan. Don't give in to distractions or let yourself procrastinate. This is your time to prepare so you'll be ready to fearlessly approach the test. Make the most of the time and stay focused.

Of course, you don't want to burn out. If you study too long you may find that you're not retaining the information very well. Take regular study breaks. For example, taking five minutes out of every hour to walk briskly, breathing deeply and swinging your arms, can help your mind stay fresh.

As you get to the end of each chapter or section, it's a good idea to do a quick review. Remind yourself of what you learned and work on any difficult parts. When you feel that you've mastered the material, move on to the next part. At the end of your study session, briefly skim through your notes again.

But while review is helpful, cramming last minute is NOT. If at all possible, work ahead so that you won't need to fit all your study into the last day. Cramming overloads your brain with more information than it can process and retain, and your tired mind may struggle to recall even previously learned information when it is overwhelmed with last-minute study. Also, the urgent nature of cramming and the stress placed on your brain contribute to anxiety. You'll be more likely to go to the test feeling unprepared and having trouble thinking clearly.

So don't cram, and don't stay up late before the test, even just to review your notes at a leisurely pace. Your brain needs rest more than it needs to go over the information again. In fact, plan to finish your studies by noon or early afternoon the day before the test. Give your brain the rest of the day to relax or focus on other things, and get a good night's sleep. Then you will be fresh for the test and better able to recall what you've studied.

Step 6: Take a practice test

Many courses offer sample tests, either online or in the study materials. This is an excellent resource to check whether you have mastered the material, as well as to prepare for the test format and environment.

Check the test format ahead of time: the number of questions, the type (multiple choice, free response, etc.), and the time limit. Then create a plan for working through them. For example, if you have 30 minutes to take a 60-question test, your limit is 30 seconds per question. Spend less time on the questions you know well so that you can take more time on the difficult ones.

If you have time to take several practice tests, take the first one open book, with no time limit. Work through the questions at your own pace and make sure you fully understand them. Gradually work up to taking a test under test conditions: sit at a desk with all study materials put away and set a timer. Pace yourself to make sure you finish the test with time to spare and go back to check your answers if you have time.

After each test, check your answers. On the questions you missed, be sure you understand why you missed them. Did you misread the question (tests can use tricky wording)? Did you forget the information? Or was it something you hadn't learned? Go back and study any shaky areas that the practice tests reveal.

Taking these tests not only helps with your grade, but also aids in combating test anxiety. If you're already used to the test conditions, you're less likely to worry about it, and working through tests until you're scoring well gives you a confidence boost. Go through the practice tests until you feel comfortable, and then you can go into the test knowing that you're ready for it.

Test Tips

On test day, you should be confident, knowing that you've prepared well and are ready to answer the questions. But aside from preparation, there are several test day strategies you can employ to maximize your performance.

First, as stated before, get a good night's sleep the night before the test (and for several nights before that, if possible). Go into the test with a fresh, alert mind rather than staying up late to study.

Try not to change too much about your normal routine on the day of the test. It's important to eat a nutritious breakfast, but if you normally don't eat breakfast at all, consider eating just a protein bar. If you're a coffee drinker, go ahead and have your normal coffee. Just make sure you time it so that the caffeine doesn't wear off right in the middle of your test. Avoid sugary beverages, and drink enough water to stay hydrated but not so much that you need a restroom break 10 minutes into the test. If your test isn't first thing in the morning, consider going for a walk or doing a light workout before the test to get your blood flowing.

Allow yourself enough time to get ready, and leave for the test with plenty of time to spare so you won't have the anxiety of scrambling to arrive in time. Another reason to be early is to select a good seat. It's helpful to sit away from doors and windows, which can be distracting. Find a good seat, get out your supplies, and settle your mind before the test begins.

When the test begins, start by going over the instructions carefully, even if you already know what to expect. Make sure you avoid any careless mistakes by following the directions.

Then begin working through the questions, pacing yourself as you've practiced. If you're not sure on an answer, don't spend too much time on it, and don't let it shake your confidence. Either skip it and come back later, or eliminate as many wrong answers as possible and guess among the remaining ones. Don't dwell on these questions as you continue—put them out of your mind and focus on what lies ahead.

Be sure to read all of the answer choices, even if you're sure the first one is the right answer. Sometimes you'll find a better one if you keep reading. But don't second-guess yourself if you do immediately know the answer. Your gut instinct is usually right. Don't let test anxiety rob you of the information you know.

If you have time at the end of the test (and if the test format allows), go back and review your answers. Be cautious about changing any, since your first instinct tends to be correct, but make sure you didn't misread any of the questions or accidentally mark the wrong answer choice. Look over any you skipped and make an educated guess.

At the end, leave the test feeling confident. You've done your best, so don't waste time worrying about your performance or wishing you could change anything. Instead, celebrate the successful completion of this test. And finally, use this test to learn how to deal with anxiety even better next time.

> **Review Video: 5 Tips to Beat Test Anxiety**
> Visit mometrix.com/academy and enter code: 570656

Important Qualification

Not all anxiety is created equal. If your test anxiety is causing major issues in your life beyond the classroom or testing center, or if you are experiencing troubling physical symptoms related to your anxiety, it may be a sign of a serious physiological or psychological condition. If this sounds like your situation, we strongly encourage you to seek professional help.

Thank You

We at Mometrix would like to extend our heartfelt thanks to you, our friend and patron, for allowing us to play a part in your journey. It is a privilege to serve people from all walks of life who are unified in their commitment to building the best future they can for themselves.

The preparation you devote to these important testing milestones may be the most valuable educational opportunity you have for making a real difference in your life. We encourage you to put your heart into it—that feeling of succeeding, overcoming, and yes, conquering will be well worth the hours you've invested.

We want to hear your story, your struggles and your successes, and if you see any opportunities for us to improve our materials so we can help others even more effectively in the future, please share that with us as well. **The team at Mometrix would be absolutely thrilled to hear from you!** So please, send us an email (support@mometrix.com) and let's stay in touch.

If you'd like some additional help, check out these other resources we offer for your exam:

http://MometrixFlashcards.com/DANB

Additional Bonus Material

Due to our efforts to try to keep this book to a manageable length, we've created a link that will give you access to all of your additional bonus material.

Please visit **https://www.mometrix.com/bonus948/danbice** to access the information.